Direct Diagnosis in Radiology

Vascular Imaging

Karl-Juergen Wolf, MD
Professor
Charité University Medical Center Berlin
Benjamin Franklin Campus
Department of Radiology
Berlin, Germany

With contributions by

Zarko Grozdanovic, Thomas Albrecht, Jens O. Heidenreich,
Andreas Schilling, Frank Wacker

250 Illustrations

Thieme
Stuttgart · New York

*Library of Congress
Cataloging-in-Publication Data*

Wolf, Karl-Jürgen.
[Gefässe. English]
Vascular imaging / Karl-Juergen Wolf ;
with contributions by Zarko Grozdanovic ...
[et al.].
  p. ; cm. – (Direct diagnosis in radiology)
Translated from the German: Gefässe /
Karl-Jürgen Wolf .... [et al.]. 2008.
Includes bibliographical references
and index.
ISBN 978-3-13-145181-1 (alk. paper)
1. Blood-vessels–Imaging–Handbooks,
manuals, etc. I. Grozdanovic, Zarko. II. Title.
III. Series: Direct diagnosis in radiology.
[DNLM: 1. Vascular Diseases–radiography–
Handbooks. WG 39 W854v 2009a]
RC691.6.I52W6513 2009
616.1'307572–dc22   2009002366

This book is an authorized and revised trans-
lation of the German edition published and
copyrighted 2007 by Georg Thieme Verlag,
Stuttgart, Germany. Title of the German
edition: Pareto-Reihe Radiologie:
Gefäße.

Translator: John Grossman, Schrepkow,
Germany

Illustrator: Karin Baum, Paphos, Cyprus

© 2009 Georg Thieme Verlag KG
Rüdigerstrasse 14, 70469 Stuttgart, Germany
http://www.thieme.de
Thieme New York, 333 Seventh Avenue,
New York, NY 10001, USA
http://www.thieme.com

Cover design: Thieme Publishing Group
Typesetting by Ziegler + Müller,
Kirchentellinsfurt, Germany
Printed by Offizin Andersen Nexö,
Zwenkau, Germany

ISBN 978-3-13-145181-1
          1 2 3 4 5 6

Important note: Medicine is an ever-chang-
ing science undergoing continual development. Research and clinical experience are
continually expanding our knowledge, in particular our knowledge of proper treatment
and drug therapy. Insofar as this book men-
tions any dosage or application, readers may
rest assured that the authors, editors, and
publishers have made every effort to ensure
that such references are in accordance with
**the state of knowledge at the time of pro-
duction of the book.**

Nevertheless, this does not involve, imply, or
express any guarantee or responsibility on
the part of the publishers in respect to any
dosage instructions and forms of applications
stated in the book. **Every user is requested to
examine carefully** the manufacturers' leaf-
lets accompanying each drug and to check, if
necessary in consultation with a physician or
specialist, whether the dosage schedules
mentioned therein or the contraindications
stated by the manufacturers differ from the
statements made in the present book. Such
examination is particularly important with
drugs that are either rarely used or have been
newly released on the market. Every dosage
schedule or every form of application used is
entirely at the user's own risk and responsibility. The authors and publishers request every
user to report to the publishers any discrepan-
cies or inaccuracies noticed. If errors in this
work are found after publication, errata will
be posted at www.thieme.com on the product
description page.

Zarko Grozdanovic, MD
Associate Professor
Charité University Medical Center Berlin
Benjamin Franklin Campus
Department of Radiology
Berlin, Germany

Thomas Albrecht, MD, FRCR
Professor
Charité University Medical Center Berlin
Benjamin Franklin Campus
Department of Radiology
Berlin, Germany

Jens O. Heidenreich, MD
Assistant Professor of Radiology
Department of Radiology
University of Louisville Hospital
Louisville, KY, USA

Andreas Schilling, MD
Institute of Radiology
Frankfurt (Oder) Medical Center
Frankfurt (Oder), Germany

Frank Wacker, MD
Professor
Charité University Medical Center Berlin
Benjamin Franklin Campus
Department of Radiology
Berlin, Germany

Acknowledgements

We would like to express our thanks to Dr. R. Klingebiel, Department of Neuroradiology, Charité University Medical Center; Dr. Ertl-Wagner, Institute of Clinical Radiology, University of Munich, Grosshadern Campus; and Dr. M. Gutberlet, Professor, Department of Diagnostic and Interventional Radiology at the Cardiac Care Center Leipzig for providing image material. We also thank Dr. S. Jovanovic, Professor, and Dr. Kostas Kandilakis, Ear, Nose, and Throat Clinic, Charité University Medical Center, Benjamin Franklin Campus, for critically reviewing portions of the manuscript.

Contents

5 Abdomen
F. Wacker, T. Albrecht

6 Kidneys
F. Wacker, Z. Grozdanovic

7 Extremities
F. Wacker, Z. Grozdanovic

3D	Three-dimensional	**HIV**	Human immunodeficiency virus
ANCA	Antineutrophil cytoplasmic antibodies	**MIP**	Maximum intensity projection
AVM	Arteriovenous malformation	**MPR**	Multiplanar reconstruction
CISS	Constructive interference in steady-state	**MRA**	Magnetic resonance angiography
CT	Computed tomography, computed tomogram	**MRI**	Magnetic resonance imaging
CTA	Computed tomography angiography	**MRV**	Magnetic resonance venography
CUP	Carcinoma of unknown primary	**P-A**	Posterior–anterior
CSF	Cerebrospinal fluid	**PTA**	Percutaneous transluminal angioplasty
DOQI	Dialysis Outcomes Quality Initiative	**PTFE**	Polytetrafluorethylene
DSA	Digital subtraction angiography	**RR**	Blood pressure according to Riva-Rocci
ECG	Electrocardiogram	**TIPS**	Transjugular intrahepatic portosystemic shunt
FDG-PET	Fluoro-18-deoxyglucose positron emission tomography	**UICC**	Union International Contre Cancer
HHT	Hereditary hemorrhagic telangiectasia		

Definition

▶ **Epidemiology**
Most common caroticobasilar anastomosis ● *Prevalence:* 0.1–0.2% of the population.

▶ **Etiology, pathophysiology, pathogenesis**
Persistent fetal anastomosis between the internal carotid and basilar artery ●
Anastomosis between the cavernous segment (C4 segment) of the internal carotid and basilar artery proximal to the origin of the posterior communicating artery ● In 25% of cases additional vascular anomalies are present ● Cerebral aneurysms are present in 10–15% of cases.

Imaging Signs

▶ **Modality of choice**
DSA.

▶ **CT findings**
Prominent artery between the internal carotid and basilar arteries.

▶ **CTA findings**
Like CT ● Additional vascular anomalies may be present.

▶ **MRI and MRA findings**
T1-weighted and T2-weighted images show the persistent trigeminal artery as a bandlike prepontine flow void between the internal carotid and basilar arteries ●
MRA confirms the diagnosis.

▶ **DSA findings**
The study demonstrates a primitive trigeminal artery supplying the distal vertebrobasilar system and the proximal hypoplastic basilar artery.

Clinical Aspects

▶ **Typical presentation**
Incidental finding.

▶ **Therapeutic options**
Incidental finding without therapeutic relevance (unless additional vascular anomalies warranting treatment are present).

▶ **Course and prognosis**
As an isolated finding, it has no clinical significance.

▶ **What does the clinician want to know?**
Exclusion of additional vascular anomalies (aneurysms in 10–15% of cases).

Fig. 1.1 a–c Primitive trigeminal artery (arrow) on MR axial T2-weighted image (**a**), MRA–MIP (**b**), and DSA (**c**). Coiled aneurysm of the anterior communicating artery (**c**) as an incidental finding.

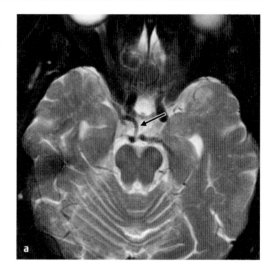

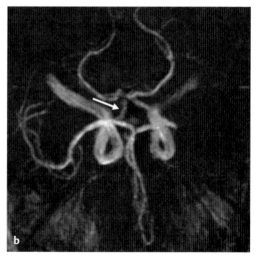

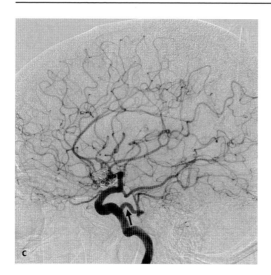

Differential Diagnosis

Persistent (primitive) hypoglossal artery	– Second most common anastomosis between the internal carotid and basilar artery
	– Anastomosis at the C1–C2 level following the bony course of the hypoglossal nerve
Persistent (primitive) otic artery	– Very rare anastomosis between the internal carotid and basilar arteries
	– Courses through the internal auditory canal
Proatlantal artery	– Anastomosis between the C2 and C3 segments of the internal carotid artery and the vertebral artery (*not* the basilar artery) at the level of C1–C2

Tips and Pitfalls

The anomalous vessel can be misinterpreted as an aneurysm of the internal carotid artery • It can be mistaken for another persistent carotid–basilar anastomosis.

Selected References

Athale SD, Jinkins JR. MRI of persistent trigeminal artery. J Comput Assist Tomogr 1993; 17: 551–554

Li MH et al. Persistent primitive trigeminal artery associated with aneurysm: Report of two cases and review of the literature. Acta Radiol 2004; 45: 664–668

Salas E et al. Persistent trigeminal artery: An anatomic study. Neurosurgery 1998; 43: 557–561

Definition

▶ **Epidemiology**
Precise information is not available.

▶ **Etiology, pathophysiology, pathogenesis**
Compression of a cranial nerve by a vascular loop in the cerebellopontine angle or the internal auditory canal ● Typically affects the trigeminal or facial nerve.

Imaging Signs

▶ **Modality of choice**
High-resolution MRI.

▶ **CT findings**
Usually normal ● Calcifying atherosclerosis can be associated with the disorder.

▶ **MRI findings**
Thin-slice T2-weighted images ● Optimal imaging can be achieved using 3T-MRI.

- Trigeminal neuralgia is most commonly caused by vascular loops formed by the superior cerebellar artery, posterior inferior cerebellar artery, or vertebro-basilar artery, in that order of occurrence.
- Facial nerve palsy is more likely to be caused by a vascular loop originating from the anterior inferior cerebellar artery than the posterior inferior cerebellar artery or vertebral artery.

▶ **DSA**
Angiography is usually not recommended as the topographic relation of vessel to nerve is not visualized.

Clinical Aspects

▶ **Typical presentation**
Trigeminal neuralgia ● Facial nerve palsy.

▶ **Therapeutic options**
Surgical (Janetta procedure) or symptomatic medical treatment.

▶ **Course and prognosis**
Postoperative long-term success rate is about 60% ● Postoperative complication rate is as high as 30%.

▶ **What does the clinician want to know?**
Verify neurovascular coupling ● Clinical correlation ● Indication for treatment ● Follow-up examination.

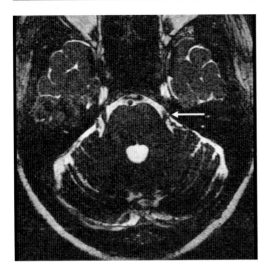

Fig. 1.2 Compressive neurovascular malformation Axial CISS sequence through the brainstem. Contact (arrow) between the trigeminal nerve and left superior cerebellar artery.

Differential Diagnosis

Vertebrobasilar dolichoectasia	– Usually in older patients with underlying atherosclerosis
Vascular malformation	– Characteristic tangle of vessels on MRI or early venous drainage
Aneurysm	– Outpouching of the arterial wall on MRI or DSA

Tips and Pitfalls

Negative MRI findings do not exclude surgical exploration.

Selected References

Chun-Cheng Q et al. A single-blinded pilot study assessing neurovascular contact by using high-resolution MR imaging in patients with trigeminal neuralgia. Eur J Radiol Nov 20, 2007 [Epub ahead of print]

Chung SS et al. Microvascular decompression of the facial nerve for the treatment of hemifacial spasm: preoperative magnetic resonance imaging related to clinical outcomes. Acta Neurochir (Wien) 2000; 142: 901–906

Holley P et al. The contribution of "time-of-flight" MRI-angiography in the study of neurovascular interactions (hemifacial spasm and trigeminal neuralgia). J Neuroradiol 1996; 23: 149–156

Papanagiotou P et al. [Vascular anomalies of the cerebellopontine angle.] Radiologe 2006; 46: 216–223 [In German]

Definition

▶ **Epidemiology**
Accounts for approximately 20% of all infratentorial and approximately 7% of all supratentorial vascular malformations ● Occasionally associated with cavernous malformations.

▶ **Etiology, pathophysiology, pathogenesis**
Circumscribed clusters of dilated capillaries interspersed with normal brain tissue ● Predilection for the brainstem, especially the pons and the deep white matter of the cerebellum and cerebral hemispheres.

Imaging Signs

▶ **Modality of choice**
MRI.

▶ **CT findings**
Normal findings.

▶ **MRI findings**
May appear as a hyperintense lesion on T2-weighted images ● Typically appears hypointense on T2*-weighted images ● Contrast-enhanced T1-weighted images show a brushlike pattern of enhancement ● Normal MRA findings.

▶ **DSA findings**
Normal findings.

Clinical Aspects

▶ **Typical presentation**
Asymptomatic incidental finding.

▶ **Therapeutic options**
No treatment is required.

▶ **Course and prognosis**
No clinical significance.

▶ **What does the clinician want to know?**
Rule out other lesions that enhance on T1-weighted sequences.

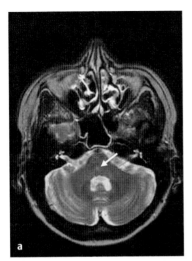

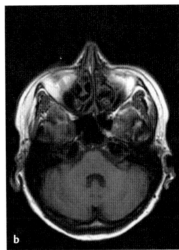

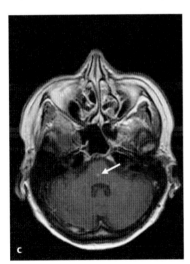

Fig. 1.3 a–c Capillary telangiectasia. Axial MR sequences through the brainstem; T2-weighted sequence (**a**), noncontrast T1-weighted sequence (**b**), and T1-weighted sequence with contrast (**c**). The telangiectasia appears hyperintense on the T2-weighted image (**a**, arrow), is not visualized on the T1-weighted sequence (**b**), and enhances homogeneously (**c**, arrow).

Differential Diagnosis

Metastasis	– History – Usually marked enhancement on T1-weighted images after contrast administration
Glioma	– Contrast pattern – Diffusion imaging, perfusion imaging, or MR spectroscopy may be indicated
Cavernous malformation	– Multiple sites – Hemosiderin rim on T2*-weighted images
Arteriovenous malformation (AVM)	– Flow voids indicative of nidus on axial T2-weighted images – Angiography shows early venous drainage – Ectatic veins

Tips and Pitfalls

Can be misinterpreted as a metastasis, glioma, cavernous malformation, or AVM.

Selected References

Castillo M et al. MR imaging and histologic features of capillary telangiectasia of the basal ganglia. AJNR Am J Neuroradiol 2001; 22: 1553–1555

Scaglione C et al. Symptomatic unruptured capillary telangiectasia of the brain stem: report of three cases and review of the literature. J Neurol Neurosurg Psychiatry 2001; 71: 390–393

Yoshida Y et al. Capillary telangiectasia of the brain stem diagnosed by susceptibility-weighted imaging. J Comput Assist Tomogr 2006; 30: 980–982

Definition

Synonyms: Cavernoma • Cavernous angioma.

▶ **Epidemiology**
Prevalence is 0.4–0.9%.

▶ **Etiology, pathophysiology, pathogenesis**
Collection of dilated sinusoidal spaces lined with endothelium and not interspersed with normal brain parenchyma (in contrast to capillary telangiectasia) • 80% of lesions are supratentorial, 20% are infratentorial, including in the brainstem • Cavernous malformations occur in familial clusters or sporadically • Multiple lesions are found in 25% of sporadic and up to 90% of familial cases.

Imaging Signs

▶ **Modality of choice**
MRI.

▶ **CT findings**
Occasionally visualized on unenhanced CT as a round to ovoid hyperdense lesion (secondary to thrombosis, hemorrhage, or calcification) • No or only slight contrast enhancement is seen.

▶ **MRI findings**
T1-weighted and T2-weighted images show an inhomogeneous focal popcorn-shaped lesion • T2-weighted images and especially T2*-weighted images show a hypointense hemosiderin rim • Inhomogeneous enhancement on enhanced T1-weighted images • Lesions are not visualized on time-of-flight MRA.

▶ **DSA findings**
Lesions are not detectable on angiography due to the slow blood flow • A cavernous malformation with hemorrhage may be indirectly visualized as a devascularized area.

Clinical Aspects

▶ **Typical presentation**
Between 38% and 55% of cases present with seizures • Focal neurological deficit • Chronic headache • Typical brainstem symptoms such as diplopia, sensory loss, or ataxia • Often asymptomatic.

▶ **Therapeutic options**
Surgery • Follow-up.

▶ **Course and prognosis**
Occasionally there is recurrent bleeding but usually without any clinically significant neurologic deficit • Life-threatening hemorrhages are rare.

▶ **What does the clinician want to know?**
Exclude other vascular diseases or tumor.

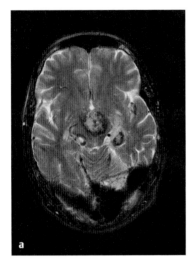

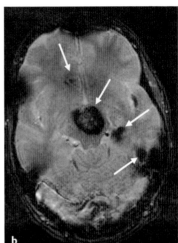

Fig. 1.4a–c Multiple cavernous malformations (arrows). Axial noncontrast T2-weighted MRI (**a**), T2*-weighted sequence (**b**), and T1-weighted sequence (**c**). T2-weighted sequence shows inhomogeneously hyperintense lesion (**a**), which on the T2*-weighted sequence appears hypointense with a pronounced hemosiderin ring (**b**). On the T1-weighted sequence portions may appear slightly hyperintense to brain tissue (**c**), consistent with small residues of hemorrhage.

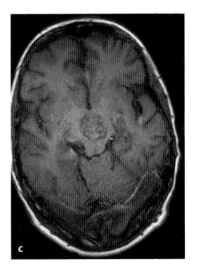

Differential Diagnosis

Oligodendroglioma — T2*-weighted sequences usually distinguish hemosiderin and calcification reliably

Tips and Pitfalls

Search for additional lesions in brainstem and spinal cord • Developmental venous anomalies can be associated with cavernous malformations.

Selected References

Abla A et al. Developmental venous anomaly, cavernous malformation, and capillary telangiectasia: spectrum of a single disease. Acta Neurochir (Wien) 2008; 150: 487–489; discussion 489.

Pozzati E et al. The neurovascular triad: Mixed cavernous, capillary, and venous malformations of the brainstem. J Neurosurg 2007; 107: 1113–1119

Wurm G et al. Cerebral cavernous malformations associated with venous anomalies: Surgical considerations. Neurosurgery 2007; 61(1 Suppl): 390–404

Wanke I et al. [Bleeding risk of intracranial vascular malformations.] Rofo 2007; 179: 365–372 [In German]

Definition

Synonym: Developmental venous anomaly.

▶ **Epidemiology**
Prevalence is 4%.

▶ **Etiology, pathophysiology, pathogenesis**
Not truly a vascular malformation, rather a variant of venous drainage • Associated with cavernous malformation in 15–20% of cases.

Imaging Signs

▶ **Modality of choice**
MRI.

▶ **CT findings**
Unenhanced CT usually normal • Contrast images show a punctate or bandlike pattern of enhancement arising from the cerebral white matter and extending to the surface of the brain.

▶ **MRI findings**
Stellate flow voids are occasionally demonstrated on T2-weighted images • T1-weighted contrast images show dilated venules deep in the white matter draining into a large transcortical collecting vein.

▶ **MRV and DSA findings**
The venous phase and MRV show the typical caput medusae pattern of fine radial venules draining into a large-caliber transcortical collecting vein.

Clinical Aspects

▶ **Typical presentation**
Usually asymptomatic • Seizures can rarely occur.

▶ **Therapeutic options**
No treatment is required.

▶ **Course and prognosis**
No clinical significance.

▶ **What does the clinician want to know?**
Exclude pathologic changes.

Differential Diagnosis

Arteriovenous malformation (AVM)	– Angiography shows early venous drainage
	– Ectatic veins
Cavernous malformation	– Multiple sites
	– Hemosiderin ring on T2*-weighted images

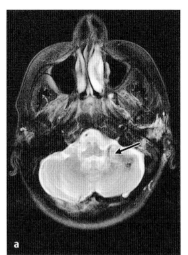

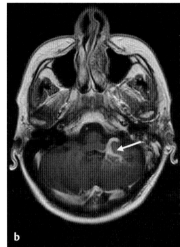

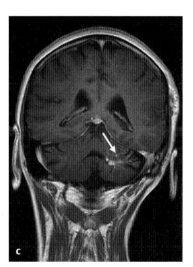

Fig. 1.5 a–c   Venous angioma. T2-weighted axial (**a**), and postcontrast T1-weighted axial (**b**) and coronal (**c**) MR images. The developmental venous anomaly appears hypointense on the T2-weighted sequences (**a**) because of a flow void. The slow venous flow produces significant enhancement on the contrast images (**b,c**), which show stellate vessels converging on a central draining vein.

Tips and Pitfalls
....

T2*-weighted MRI sequences should be obtained to evaluate for associated cavernous malformations.

Selected References

Lasjaunias P et al. Developmental venous anomalies (DVA): The so-called venous angioma. Neurosurg Rev 1986; 9: 233–242

Lee C et al. MR evaluation of developmental venous anomalies: Medullary venous anatomy of venous angiomas. AJNR Am J Neuroradiol 1996; 17: 61–70

Peebles TR, Vieco PT. Intracranial developmental venous anomalies: Diagnosis using CT angiography. J Comput Assist Tomogr 1997; 21: 582–586

Definition

▶ **Epidemiology**
Extremely rare • Accounts for less than 1% of all congenital cardiovascular disorders • Males are more often affected than females.

▶ **Etiology, pathophysiology, pathogenesis**
Central AVM draining into the aneurysmally dilated vein of Galen • The high shunt volume often leads to cardiac failure in newborns.

Imaging Signs

▶ **Modality of choice**
MRI, MRA.

▶ **CT findings**
Significantly dilated vein of Galen • Often there is severe internal hydrocephalus with periventricular leukoencephalopathy • Intracerebral or intraventricular hemorrhages occasionally occur • Malformation enhances with contrast.

▶ **MRI findings**
  – T2-weighted images: Flow void in dilated vein • Internal hydrocephalus with hyperintense periventricular CSF diapedesis.
  – T1-weighted images: Demonstrate the structure of the malformation in greater detail.
  – MRA: Arterial feeders • Venous drainage.

▶ **DSA**
Only prior to intervention • Super-selective contrast injection prior to embolization is recommended.

Clinical Aspects

▶ **Typical presentation**
The shunt volume and the resulting high cardiac output lead to fetal hydrocephalus. • Newborn present with heart failure.

▶ **Therapeutic options**
Glue embolization (often multiple) • Management of the cardiac insufficiency.

▶ **Course and prognosis**
Fatal if left untreated • Prognosis after successful treatment depends on the extent of the brain damage.

▶ **What does the clinician want to know?**
Rule out other malformations • Extent of brain damage.

Differential Diagnosis

Childhood: Dural arteriovenous fistula • AVM • Other systemic AVM with high shunt volume, such as hepatic or pulmonary shunt.

Fig. 1.6a,b Vein of Galen malformation. DSA: P-A (**a**) and lateral (**b**) views. Extensive tangle of vessels with early arterial drainage into the ectatic vein of Galen.

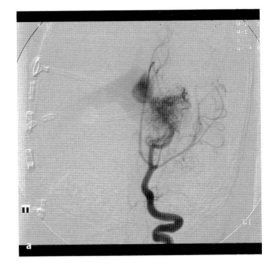

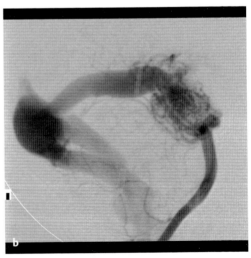

Tips and Pitfalls

Treatment of hydrocephalus without embolization of arteriovenous fistula is insufficient ● Can be misinterpreted as a cystic tumor on prenatal ultrasound.

Selected References

Chooi WK et al. Assessment of blood supply to intracranial pathologies in children using MR digital subtraction angiography. Pediatr Radiol 2006; 36: 1057–1062

Landis MS. Vein of Galen malformation. CMAJ 2006; 175: 1059

Lasjaunias PL et al. The management of vein of Galen aneurysmal malformations. Neurosurgery 2006; 59 (Suppl 3): 184–194

Definition

Synonym: Referred to as angioma in older literature.

▶ **Epidemiology**

Most common symptomatic vascular malformation ● *Prevalence:* 5–15 : 100 000 ● Clinical manifestation in early adulthood, typically between the ages of 20 and 40 ● Although congenital, it rarely gets diagnosed in children ● Males and females are affected equally often ● *Location:* 85% supratentorial, 15% posterior cranial fossa ● 98% of cases are sporadic.

▶ **Etiology, pathophysiology, pathogenesis**

Uncertain ● Dysregulation of angiogenesis at the level of vascular endothelial growth factors and their receptors has been postulated ● Characteristic findings include shunts between cerebral arteries and draining veins with multiple fistulas ● Occasionally associated with flow-related extranidal or intranidal aneurysms.

Imaging Signs

▶ **Modality of choice**

CT and MRI in the acute phase ● Gold standard prior to treatment is DSA.

▶ **CT findings**

Reliably demonstrates intracranial hemorrhage and complications ● Hemorrhage can completely compress the AVM ● Findings in nonhemorrhagic cases include tortuous, ectatic vessels that are isodense or hypodense to surrounding brain tissue ● Vascular calcifications are present in 25–30% of cases ● Pronounced enhancement is found in ectatic vessels.

▶ **MRI findings**

Characteristic flow signals (tortuous flow voids) on T1-weighted and T2-weighted sequences ● Hemosiderin, deoxyhemoglobin or methemoglobin on T1-weighted and T2*-weighted sequences ● Hyperintense gliosis in surrounding tissue on T2-weighted and FLAIR sequences.

▶ **MRA**

Evaluation of vascular structures is possible only to a limited extent.

▶ **DSA findings**

Gold standard for evaluating vascular architecture, size of the nidus, flow-related aneurysms (present in 15–20% of cases), venous drainage, and high-flow fistulas ● Typically performed simultaneously with endovascular therapy.

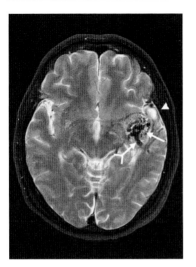

Fig. 1.7 Cerebral AVM. Axial T2-weighted MR image. Part of the nidus (arrow) is recognizable as a nodular hypointensity resulting from the flow void and drainage into the hypointense ectatic veins (forked arrow). Adjacent to this is a small triangular defect secondary to hemorrhage, appearing hyperintense on the T2-weighted sequence.

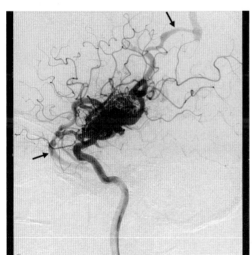

Fig. 1.8 Lateral DSA of the arteriovenous malformation. The nidus and draining ectatic cortical (arrows) veins are visualized.

Fig. 1.9 Superselective visualization of a portion of the nidus with early arterial drainage into the ectatic veins.

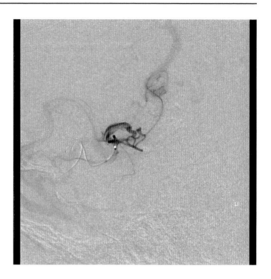

Clinical Aspects

▶ **Typical presentation**
   Cerebral hemorrhage (50% of cases) • Seizure (25% of cases) • Focal neurologic findings (25% of cases) • Headache (25% of cases).
   – Spetzler–Martin classification to estimate surgical risk:
   – *Size:* < 3 cm, 3–6 cm, > 6 cm.
   – *Location of the lesion:* Crucial or noncrucial region of the brain.
   – *Venous drainage:* Deep and/or superficial.
▶ **Therapeutic options**
   – *Acute:* Symptomatic treatment of cerebral hemorrhage and seizures.
   – *After resorption of or in the absence of hemorrhage:* Endovascular embolization • Surgical resection • Radiation therapy with the goal to avoid hemorrhage or recurrent hemorrhage may be indicated • Purely symptomatic therapy of AVM associated symptoms.
▶ **Course and prognosis**
   AVMs are dynamic lesions that can spontaneously change size • Spontaneous remissions are rare • Left untreated, there is a lifelong risk of hemorrhage which is increased once a hemorrhage has already occurred • The annual risk of recurrent hemorrhage is estimated at 2–10%.
▶ **What does the clinician want to know?**
   Size • Location • Venous drainage • Flow-related aneurysms • Hemorrhage • High-flow fistula.

Differential Diagnosis

Cavernous angioma	– Slight or absent contrast enhancement
	– Small grapelike lesions
Dural AVM	– DSA shows involvement of dural branches
Low-grade gliomas	– Slight enhancement

Tips and Pitfalls

Complete compression of vascular structures secondary to intracranial hemorrhage can mask the AVM • AVM should be excluded especially where intraparenchymal hemorrhage occurs in young adults.

Selected References

Byrne JV. Cerebrovascular malformations. Eur Radiol 2005; 15: 448–452

Heidenreich JO et al. Bleeding complications after endovascular therapy of cerebral arteriovenous malformations. AJNR Am J Neuroradiol 2006; 27: 313–316

Hofmeister C et al. Demographic, morphological, and clinical characteristics of 1289 patients with brain arteriovenous malformation. Stroke 2000; 31: 1307–1310

Stapf C et al. Predictors of hemorrhage in patients with untreated brain arteriovenous malformation. Neurology 2006; 66: 1350–1355

Definition

Synonyms: Dural arteriovenous fistula • Dural fistula.

▶ **Epidemiology**
Accounts for 10–15% of all intracranial vascular malformations.

▶ **Etiology, pathophysiology, pathogenesis**
Often acquired • Existing microscopic anastomoses open between the arterial and venous vascular tracts or angiogenesis occurs in the dura mater because of altered arteriovenous pressure gradients • Accompanied by development of venous anomalies due to venous thrombosis, traumatic head injury, or transcranial surgery • Arterial inflow via meningeal branches • Drainage occurs through dural sinuses or cortical veins • Often combined with stenosis or occlusion of the draining dural sinus.

Imaging Signs

▶ **Modality of choice**
DSA • MRI • MRA.

▶ **CT findings**
Often normal • Findings may include enlarged dural sinus and tortuous cortical veins.

▶ **MRI findings**
Often normal • Findings of sinus thrombosis (direct visualization of T2 hyperintense thrombus) • Flow signal in cortical veins or sinus from microfistulas.

▶ **DSA findings**
Meningeal arteries feed the dural AVM • The dural AVM drains through cortical veins • Internal carotid artery–cavernous sinus fistula represents a special type of dural arteriovenous fistula.

Clinical Aspects

▶ **Typical presentation**
This depends on age, location, and severity of the dural AVM • Pulsatile tinnitus • Cranial nerve palsy • Chemosis • Optic atrophy • Optic disk edema • Headache • Signs of elevated cranial pressure such as nausea and vomiting • Seizures • Focal neurologic deficit • Dementia • Involvement of leptomeningeal veins increases risk of hemorrhage.

▶ **Therapeutic options**
Endovascular therapy • Stereotactic radiation • Surgical resection.

▶ **Course and prognosis**
Spontaneous occlusion rarely occurs • Variable course • Symptoms usually remit completely after successful occlusion although recurrence is common, especially with incomplete occlusion • Subdural or intraparenchymal hemorrhage may result in permanent neurological deficits.

▶ **What does the clinician want to know?**
Rule out AVM • Determine cause of tinnitus • Risk of particle embolization.

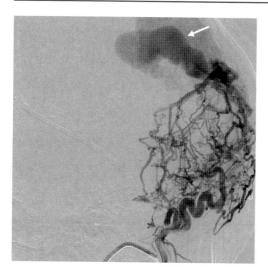

Fig. 1.10 Dural AVM. DSA shows extensive nidus supplied by branches of the occipital artery and draining into ectatic cortical veins (arrow).

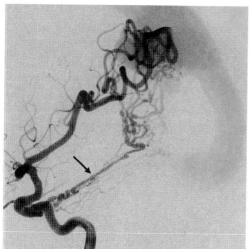

Fig. 1.11 Tentorial dural AVM. DSA demonstrates that it is supplied by a meningeal branch of the internal carotid artery (arrow).

Differential Diagnosis

Glomus tumor (paraganglioma)	– Pronounced tumor blush on DSA
Cerebral AVM	– Fed by cerebral, not dural arteries

Tips and Pitfalls

Missing out on dural feeders can lead to misdiagnosis as proper AVM ● Overlooking anastomoses between the internal carotid and external carotid circulation is another error.

Selected References

Kim MS et al. Clinical characteristics of dural arteriovenous fistula. J Clin Neurosci 2002; 9: 147–155

Kwon BJ et al. MR imaging findings of intracranial dural arteriovenous fistulas: relations with venous drainage patterns. AJNR Am J Neuroradiol 2005; 26: 2500–2507

Luciani A et al. Spontaneous closure of dural arteriovenous fistulas: report of three cases and review of the literature. AJNR Am J Neuroradiol 2001; 22: 992–996

Shownkeen H et al. Endovascular treatment of transverse-sigmoid sinus dural arteriovenous malformations presenting as pulsatile tinnitus. Skull Base 2001; 11: 13–23

Definition

Synonym: Caroticocavernous fistula.

▶ **Epidemiology**
Spontaneous or traumatic • Accounts for about 12% of all intracranial fistulas.

▶ **Etiology, pathophysiology, pathogenesis**
Special type of dural arteriovenous fistula • High-flow fistula between the cavernous segment of the internal carotid and the cavernous sinus itself.

Imaging Signs

▶ **Modality of choice**
MRI • DSA.

▶ **CT findings**
Exophthalmos • Findings occasionally include prominent cortical veins • Subarachnoid hemorrhage from reflux into cortical veins with subsequent rupture • Contrast images show a dilated superior ophthalmic vein and greatly enlarged cavernous sinus.

▶ **MRI findings**
Flow void in the cavernous sinus and in the dilated ophthalmic vein • Arterial time-of-flight angiography shows a prominent ophthalmic vein.

▶ **DSA findings**
Rapid filling of the enlarged cavernous sinus after injection of contrast into the internal carotid artery • Drainage is usually via one or both superior ophthalmic veins into the facial vein • Alternatively, drainage may be via the superior and inferior petrosal sinuses into the internal jugular vein or via the basal vein of Rosenthal into the vein of Galen.

Clinical Aspects

▶ **Typical presentation**
Pulsatile exophthalmos • Loss of visual acuity • Conjunctival inflammation and injection.

▶ **Therapeutic options**
Endovascular occlusion of the fistula with platinum coils or balloons • When all else fails, occlusion of the internal carotid artery.

▶ **Course and prognosis**
Spontaneous occlusion is rare • Progression of symptoms in untreated cases.

▶ **What does the clinician want to know?**
Identify the fistula and demonstrate the venous drainage pathways.

Fig. 1.12 a, b Carotico-cavernous fistula. DSA, P-A (**a**) and lateral (**b**) view. Early arterial filling (arrow marks the internal carotid artery) of the cavernous sinus (forked arrow), draining into both petrosal sinuses. Ectatic superior ophthalmic vein (arrowhead).

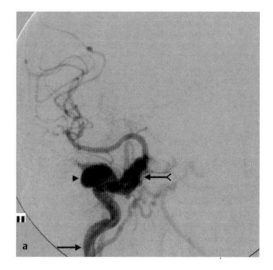

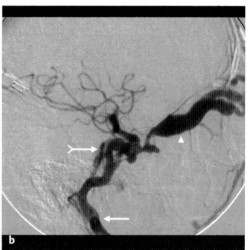

Differential Diagnosis

Thyroid ophthalmopathy	– Bilateral in 80% of cases – Hyperthyroidism in 70% of cases
Thrombosis or thrombophlebitis of the cavernous sinus	– Central contrast enhancement – No flow voids – May occur in addition to caroticocavernous fistula
Orbital pseudotumor	– Idiopathic, inflammatory, responds to steroids

Tips and Pitfalls

Failure to pay attention to the orbits when interpreting cranial CT studies.

Selected References

Andres RH et al. [Diagnosis and treatment of carotid cavernous fistulas.] Rofo 2008; 180: 604–613 [In German]

Chen CC et al. CT angiography and MR angiography in the evaluation of carotid cavernous sinus fistula prior to embolization: A comparison of techniques. AJNR Am J Neuroradiol 2005; 26: 2349–2356

Hähnel S et al. [Injury of craniocervical arteries: Imaging findings and therapy.] Fortschr Röntgenstr 2007; 179: 119–129 [In German]

Definition

▶ **Epidemiology**
  Prevalence is 2 : 100 000.
▶ **Etiology, pathophysiology, pathogenesis**
  Sporadic congenital malformation ● The embryonic cortical veins fail to regress ● This produces deep venous occlusion and venous stasis ● This in turn leads to cortical anoxia.

Imaging Signs

▶ **Modality of choice**
  CT ● MRI ● DSA.
▶ **CT findings**
  – *Early stage:* Cortical calcifications resembling railroad tracks beginning in the occipital and parietal regions.
  – *Late stage:* Severe cortical calcifications ● Beginning in the cortical region ● Dilation of the adjacent frontal sinus ● Widening of the diploe of the skull.
▶ **MRI findings**
  – *Early stage:* Significant area enhancement of the angioma of the pia mater throughout the affected subarachnoid space.
  – *Late stage:* Decreased enhancement because of calcification ● Cortical atrophy ● Prominent choroid plexus after contrast administration ● Prominent subependymal and medullary veins ● Reduced cortical veins.
▶ **DSA findings**
  Marked meningeal enhancement due to the angioma of the pia mater ● Reduced cortical draining veins.

Clinical Aspects

▶ **Typical presentation**
  Port wine facial nevus (in 98% of cases in the area supplied by the first trigeminal branch) ● Mental retardation ● Epileptic seizures (90% of cases) ● Hemiplegia ● Hemianopia ● Buphthalmos ● Glaucoma.
▶ **Therapeutic options**
  Symptomatic treatment.
▶ **Course and prognosis**
  Progressive epileptic seizures ● Increasing neurologic deficits.
▶ **What does the clinician want to know?**
  Differentiate from other vascular malformations.

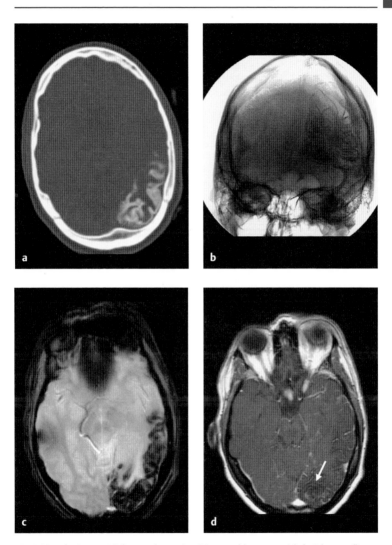

Fig. 1.13 a–d   Sturge–Weber syndrome in a 23-year-old woman with facial nevus flammeus and epileptic seizures. Unenhanced cranial CT (**a**). Gyrate calcifications tracing the band of the cortex. DSA mask, also showing gyrate calcifications in the angioma (**b**). MR T2*-weighted sequence (**c**). Significant signal voids in the affected gyri. MR T1-weighted image after contrast administration (**d**). Enhancement in the subpial angioma (arrow) (with the courtesy of Dr. Ertl-Wagner, Munich).

Differential Diagnosis

Klippel–Trenaunay syndrome	– Cutaneous angioma – Soft tissue and/or bone hypertrophy – Leptomeningeal vascular malformation
Wyburn–Mason syndrome	– Nevus – AVM arising from the retina and involving the entire visual pathway

Selected References

Benedikt RA et al. Sturge–Weber syndrome: cranial MR imaging with Gd-DTPA. AJNR Am J Neuroradiol 1993; 14: 409–415

Ertl-Wagner B. Pädiatrische Neuroradiologie. Berlin: Springer; 2007

Vilela PF. Sturge–Weber syndrome revisited. Evaluation of encephalic morphological changes with computerized tomography and magnetic resonance. Acta Med Port 2003; 16: 141–148

Definition

▶ **Epidemiology**
Sporadic in 75% of cases ● Increased familial incidence in 25% of cases (von Hippel–Lindau disease) ● Accounts for 2% of all primary CNS tumors ● Most common cerebellar tumor in adults ● Rarely in the supratentorial region, but in those cases occurring along the visual pathway ● Accounts for 5–15% of all spinal cord tumors.

▶ **Etiology, pathophysiology, pathogenesis**
Benign, slow-growing solid or cystic tumor arising from mesodermal tissue ● Occurs primarily in the cerebellar hemispheres, less often in the brainstem and only rarely in the cerebrum ● Compression of the fourth ventricle can occur, leading to hydrocephalus.

Imaging Signs

▶ **Modality of choice**
MRI.

▶ **CT findings**
Round, sharply demarcated hypodense areas ● Contrast-enhanced images may demonstrate a hyperdense halo ● The angiomatous portion often appears as an enhancing nodule on the margin of a cystic formation.

▶ **MRI findings**
More sensitive than CT for smaller hemangioblastomas ● Hyperintense round structure ● T1-weighted images show a round hypointensity with nodules that enhance markedly.

▶ **DSA findings**
Round, nonvascularized mass with hypervascularized nodule exhibiting persistent filling until the late venous phase ● Dilated arterial feeders and draining veins.

Clinical Aspects

▶ **Typical presentation**
Patients are typically 40–60 years old ● Headache (85% of cases) ● Vomiting and nausea ● Gait disturbances and equilibrium problems ● Sporadic form occasionally includes elevated erythropoietin with secondary polycythemia.

▶ **Therapeutic options**
Surgical resection ● Preoperative embolization is indicated only under certain conditions due to the high rate of postinterventional bleeding.

▶ **Course and prognosis**
Benign slow-growing tumor ● Potentially curable ● Additional lesions develop in von Hippel–Lindau syndrome ● 10-year survival rate is 85% ● Rate of recurrence is 15–20%.

Fig. 1.14 Hemangioblastoma. MR T1-weighted image after contrast administration. Typical cystic form of hemangioblastoma. Nidus enhances markedly.

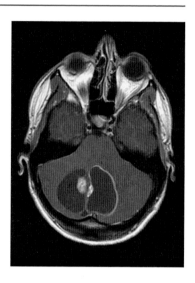

▶ **What does the clinician want to know?**
Exclude other tumors, especially metastases ● Evaluate other lesions in the familial form (von Hippel–Lindau syndrome)—retina (hemangioblastoma), kidneys (hypernephroma), adrenal glands (pheochromocytoma), bladder (cystadenoma).

Differential Diagnosis

Pilocytic astrocytoma	– Enhances only shortly on angiography
Arachnoid cysts of the posterior cranial fossa	– No enhancing margin
Metastasis	– Usually less vascularized
Glioma	– No early venous drainage
Clear-cell ependymoma	– No early venous drainage

Tips and Pitfalls

Can be misinterpreted as a metastasis.

Selected References

Kuhne M et al. Challenging manifestations of malignancies. Polycythemia and high serum erythropoietin level as a result of hemangioblastoma. J Clin Oncol 2004; 22: 3639–3640

Peker S et al. Suprasellar haemangioblastoma. Report of two cases and review of the literature. J Clin Neurosci 2005; 12: 85–89

Wierzba-Bobrowicz T et al. Haemangioblastoma of the posterior cranial fossa: Clinico-neuropathological study. Folia Neuropathol 2003; 41: 245–249

Definition

Synonym: Cerebellar and retinal angiomatosis.
- ► **Epidemiology**
  Prevalence: 1 : 30 000–50 000.
- ► **Etiology, pathophysiology, pathogenesis**
  Cerebellar hemangioblastoma and retinal angioma ● Autosomal dominant tumor syndrome with hemangioblastoma, hypernephroma, cystadenoma, and pheochromocytoma ● *Distribution:* 50 % in the spinal cord, 35–40 % in the cerebellum, 10 % in the brainstem, 1 % in the supratentorial region.

Imaging Signs

- ► **Modality of choice**
  MRI.
- ► **CT findings**
  Two-thirds of cases involve sharply demarcated cysts and nodules in the cerebellum ● One-third involve solid lesions ● Obstructive hydrocephalus may be present ● Marked enhancement.
- ► **MRI findings**
  - T2-weighted images: Hyperintense cyst ● Hypointense nodulus.
  - T1-weighted images: Hypointense cyst ● Nodule is isointense to soft tissue ● Nodules show intense homogenous enhancement.
- ► **DSA findings**
  Highly vascularized mass.

Clinical Aspects

- ► **Typical presentation**
  Early symptoms often involve the eyes (retinal hemangioblastoma) ● Hemangioblastomas have several growth periods interspersed with steady phases ● Neurologic symptoms vary according to location.
- ► **Therapeutic options**
  Surgery.
- ► **Course and prognosis**
  Disease tends to progress ● Annual MRI follow-up studies of the central nervous system are required.
- ► **What does the clinician want to know?**
  Extent of the disorder.

Fig. 1.15 Von Hippel–Lindau syndrome. MRI. Multiple cerebellar hemangioblastomas.

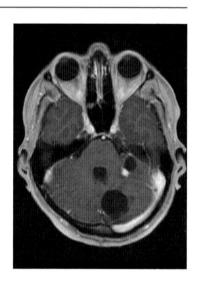

Differential Diagnosis

Hypervascular metastases
– History
– Possible history of CUP syndrome

Solitary hemangioblastoma
– Genotyping

Pilocytic astrocytoma
– Follow-up
– Biopsy

Multiple AVMs in vascular neurocutaneous syndrome
– Early venous filling on DSA

Tips and Pitfalls

Can be misinterpreted as one of the other disorders considered in differential diagnosis.

Selected References

Couch V et al. von Hippel-Lindau disease. Mayo Clin Proc 2000; 75: 265–272

Hes FJ, Feldberg MA. Von Hippel-Lindau disease: Strategies in early detection (renal-, adrenal-, pancreatic masses). Eur Radiol 1999; 9: 598–610

Definition

▶ **Etiology, pathophysiology, pathogenesis**
  Inflammation of arteries with or without necrosis of the vascular wall of widely varying etiology ● Infectious and noninfectious causes have been identified:
  – Infectious form: Bacterial ● Tuberculous ● Mycotic ● Viral ● Syphilitic.
  – Polyarteritis nodosa.
  – Cell-mediated: Giant-cell arteritis, Takayasu arteritis ● Temporal arteritis (giant cell arteritis).
  – Granulomatous angiitis: Primary central nervous system angiitis ● Wegener granulomatosis ● Sarcoid.
  – Collagen diseases.
  – Caused by medications or other drugs: Ergotamines ● Amphetamines ● Heroin ● Cocaine.
  – From radiation.

Imaging Signs

Characteristics: Irregularities in vascular caliber ● Stenoses ● Occlusion ● Aneurysms.

▶ **Modality of choice**
  MRI ● Where spatial resolution is limited, MRI is used for screening ● Conventional DSA.

▶ **CT findings**
  Can be normal ● Reduced density in the basal ganglia and subcortical region.

▶ **MRI findings**
  – T2-weighted images: Multilocular hyperintensities especially along the corticomedullary junction.
  – T1-weighted images: Multilocular defects of the blood–brain barrier may be visible after contrast administration.

▶ **DSA findings**
  Multiple short stenoses and constrictions ● Vascular dilations alternate with areas where the vessel is not visualized.

Clinical Aspects

▶ **Typical presentation**
  Headache ● Multifocal neurologic deficits ● Encephalopathy ● Infarction ● When vasculitis is clinically suspected, laboratory tests, spinal tap, and imaging (possibly including catheter angiography) are indicated ● Diagnosis can only be confirmed by histologic studies.

▶ **Therapeutic options**
  This depends on the etiology ● Often a combination of immunosuppressants may be used.

Fig. 1.16 a, b   Intracranial vasculitis. Arterial time-of-flight MRA showing abrupt change in caliber (see arrow).

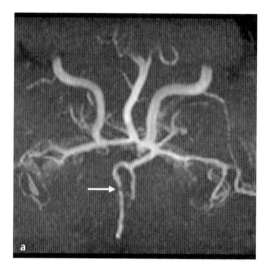

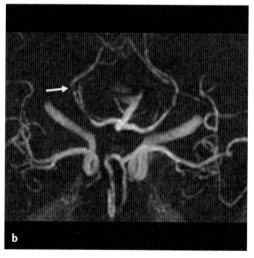

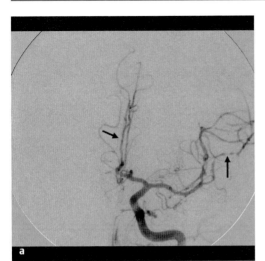

Fig. 1.17 a, b DSA. Typical abrupt changes in caliber (arrows) in the affected arteries are visible.

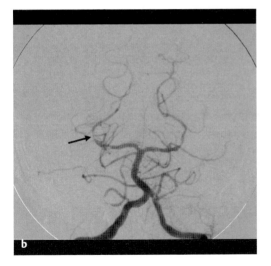

► **Course and prognosis**
This depends on the etiology ● Complete recovery is possible ● Residues of cerebral infarcts may persist ● Course may be progressive with additional insults.

► **What does the clinician want to know?**
Rule out atherosclerosis.

Differential Diagnosis

Vasospasms	– History of subarachnoid hemorrhage
Intracranial occlusive arterial disease	– Older patient
	– Diabetes mellitus
	– Vascular calcification
Intracranial atherosclerosis	– Vascular calcification

Tips and Pitfalls

Imaging studies can be normal ● It is crucial to correlate imaging findings with clinical and laboratory findings ● Can be misinterpreted as an intracranial atherosclerosis.

Selected References

Kuker W. Cerebral vasculitis: Imaging signs revisited. Neuroradiology 2007; 49: 471–479
Scolding NJ, EFNS Cerebral Vasculitis Task Force. The recognition, diagnosis and management of cerebral vasculitis: A European survey. Eur J Neurol 2002; 9: 343–347
Wasserman BA et al. Reliability of normal findings on MR imaging for excluding the diagnosis of vasculitis of the central nervous system. AJR Am J Roentgenol 2001; 177: 455–459

Definition

Synonym: Japanese for "cloud of smoke."

▶ **Epidemiology**
Most commonly seen in Japanese children and in children of African descent with sickle-cell anemia.

▶ **Etiology, pathophysiology, pathogenesis**
Idiopathic progressive infantile arteriopathy ● Onset of symptoms is often in childhood or adolescence ● Usually multiple ischemic episodes occur ● Clinical findings and course depend on the speed and extent of the occlusions and on the effectiveness of collateral circulation ● *Causes are numerous:* Idiopathic, genetic, inflammatory, congenital mesenchymal defect, premature aging syndrome.

Imaging Signs

▶ **Modality of choice**
DSA.

▶ **CT findings**
Primarily frontal atrophy occurs in up to 60% of cases in children ● Cerebral bleeding occurs in adults ● Punctate enhancement in the basal ganglia is seen after contrast administration.

▶ **MRI findings**
– T2-weighted images: Hyperintense areas from infarctions of minor vessels in the cortex and white matter.
– T1-weighted images: Multiple punctate hyperintensities in the basal ganglia ● Marked enhancement after contrast administration.
– MRA: Branches of the middle cerebral artery are not visualized.

▶ **DSA findings**
"Cloud of smoke."
– *Early phase:* Stenoses in the M1, A1, and P1 segments or in the distal internal carotid artery.
– *Advanced stage:* Collaterals arising from the deep perforating branches of the middle cerebral artery.
– *Late stage:* Transdural collaterals arising from meningeal branches.

Clinical Aspects

▶ **Typical presentation**
Ischemia (transient ischemic attack, infarction) in children ● Hemorrhage (subarachnoid or intraventricular) in adults.

▶ **Therapeutic options**
External carotid artery/internal carotid artery (ECA/ICA) bypass ● Surgical neutralization of the sympathetic nerve (ganglionectomy of the superior cervical ganglion or perivascular sympathectomy).

Fig. 1.18 a–d Moya-moya disease. DSA. Early arterial phase (**a, b**). Area supplied by the middle cerebral artery abruptly terminates proximally in the M1 segment (arrow), continuing only in a veil-like pattern of small-caliber arteries.

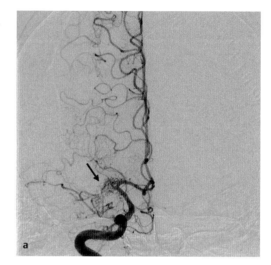

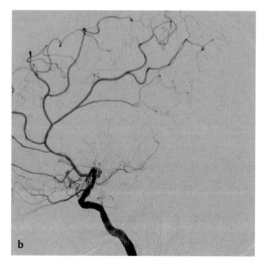

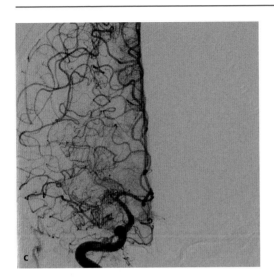

Late arterial phase (**c, d**). Partial filling of the area supplied by the middle cerebral artery from the territory of the anterior cerebral artery.

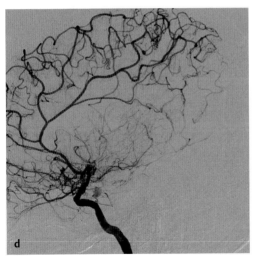

▶ **Course and prognosis**

Progressive stenoses leading to increasing ischemic and hemorrhagic insults ● Prognosis tends to be unfavorable but depends on stage of the disease and the patient's age.

▶ **What does the clinician want to know?**

Extent of vascular involvement ● Differentiate from other vascular disorders.

Differential Diagnosis

Dissection	– Spontaneous
	– Trauma
	– Idiopathic
	– Infectious
Vasospasm	– Subarachnoid hemorrhage
	– Infectious
	– Idiopathic
Vascular encasement by tumor	– Pituitary adenoma
	– Craniopharyngioma

Tips and Pitfalls

Can be misinterpreted as one of the other disorders considered in differential diagnosis.

Selected References

Ganesan V et al. Conventional cerebral angiography in children with ischemic stroke. Pediatr Neurol 1999; 20: 38–42

Horn P et al. [Spontaneous occlusion of the circle of Willis (moyamoya disease). Diagnosis and therapy.] Nervenarzt 2001; 72: 406–415 [In German]

Papanagiotou P et al. [Moyamoya disease.] Radiologe 2005; 45: 466–470 [In German]

Definition

▶ **Epidemiology**
Hypercoagulability is responsible for up to 50% of all ischemic strokes in children under 15 years ● Dissection and atheromatous plaques are more common in adolescents.

▶ **Etiology, pathophysiology, pathogenesis**
  – Cardiac causes, left-to-right shunt.
  – Birth trauma.
  – Neurocutaneous syndrome (neurofibromatosis, tuberous sclerosis).
  – *Vasculopathy:* Chickenpox ● Systemic angiitis (Takayasu, Kawasaki, Moyamoya disease, polyarteritis nodosa).
  – *Hypercoagulability:* Congenital coagulation disorder (factor V Leiden deficiency) ● Acquired coagulation disorder with hypercoagulability (such as leukemia).
  – *Adolescents:* Drug use ● Oral contraceptives.

Imaging Signs

▶ **Modality of choice**
MRI ● CT.

▶ **CT and CTA findings**
Employed to exclude hemorrhage ● Evaluation of sinus thrombosis (delta sign, empty triangle sign) ● Evaluation of cerebral perfusion ● *Caution:* Involves exposure to ionizing radiation.

▶ **MRI findings**
  – T2-weighted images: Hyperintense signal in the affected areas ● Caution: In very small children, normal mature white matter is primarily hyperintense, whereas the ischemic tissue tends to be hypointense.
  – T1-weighted images: Normal findings.
  – T2*-weighted images: Exclude hemorrhage.
  – Diffusion-weighted images: Diffusion restriction.

▶ **DSA**
Usually not indicated, but may help to clarify etiology.

Clinical Aspects

▶ **Typical presentation**
This depends on the extent and location ● Seizures in newborns and infants, delayed development, poor feeding.

▶ **Therapeutic options**
Causal or symptomatic, depending on the etiology ● Immunosuppression ● Rehabilitation.

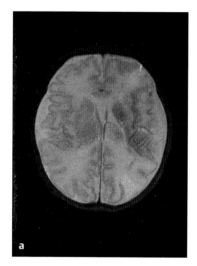
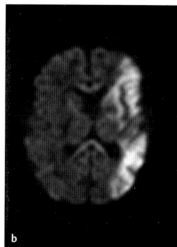

Fig. 1.19a–c Ischemic insult in the territory of the middle cerebral artery in a child. Axial MR T2-weighted image (**a**). Infarcted area is difficult to distinguish from the hyperintense immature white matter. Diffusion weighted image (**b**). The two component middle cerebral artery infarcts are readily demarcated as hyperintense areas. T1-weighted image (**c**). The infarcted areas are more readily demarcated (hypointense to parenchyma).

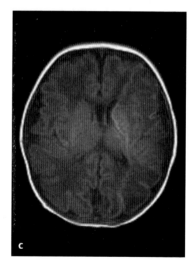

▶ **Course and prognosis**
This depends on the extent and location and on management of a possible underlying disorder ● Prognosis is better for children than for adults (due to plasticity of the brain).

▶ **What does the clinician want to know?**
Etiology ● Therapeutic options ● Prognosis.

Differential Diagnosis

Seizures from other causes – Malformations
– Masses
– Impaired cortical development

Tips and Pitfalls

Underestimating the size of the infarcted area.

Selected References

Atkinson DS. Computed tomography of pediatric stroke. Semin Ultrasound CT MR 2006; 27: 207–218

Blankenberg FG et al. Neonatal intracranial ischemia and hemorrhage: diagnosis with US, CT, and MR imaging. Radiology 1996; 199: 253–259

Wu YW et al. Perinatal arterial stroke: understanding mechanisms and outcomes. Semin Neurol 2005; 25: 424–434

Definition

▶ **Epidemiology**
Accounts for 1% of strokes ● Responsible for up to 20% of the primary intraparenchymal hemorrhages in patients over 60 years ● Often occurs in Alzheimer disease (over 80% of cases) and Down syndrome ● Autopsy finding in up to 30% of healthy elderly patients.

▶ **Etiology, pathophysiology, pathogenesis**
Idiopathic or secondary and reactive (as in chronic dialysis or chronic infection) ● Amyloidosis is a rare disorder caused by extracellular deposition of amyloid ● Amyloid deposits lead to microangiopathy ● In patients with normal blood pressure, this leads to chronic lobar hemorrhages of varying age (subcortical, usually parietal or occipital, less often in the brainstem or basal ganglia).

Imaging Signs

▶ **Modality of choice**
MRI.

▶ **CT findings**
Cortical and/or subcortical hemorrhages with irregular margins ● Surrounding edema ● Can expand into the subarachnoid or intraventricular space ● Does not enhance except in the rare case of an amyloidoma.

▶ **MRI findings**
– T1 and T2*-weighted images: Hypointense or isointense hematoma ● One-third of lesions are chronic multifocal "black dots" consistent with hemosiderin deposits ● In 70% of cases, there are associated focal or confluent white matter disorders.
– T1-weighted images: Findings depend on the age of the hemorrhage ● Initially hypointense ● Later hyperintense.

▶ **DSA findings**
Findings are normal or show effects of nonvascularized mass.

Clinical Aspects

▶ **Typical presentation**
Stroke due to acute hemorrhage ● Dementia.

▶ **Therapeutic options**
None ● Surgical removal of hematoma where indicated.

▶ **Course and prognosis**
Progressive symptoms.

▶ **What does the clinician want to know?**
Exclude other types of hemorrhage.

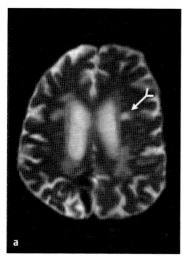

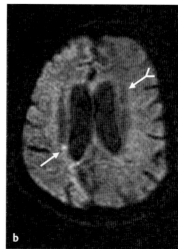

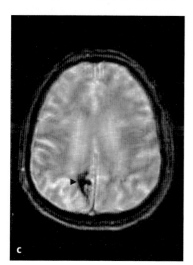

Fig. 1.20 a–c Cerebral amyloid angiopathy. MR diffusion weighted image (b = 0) (**a**). Diffusion weighted image (b = 1000) (**b**). T2*-weighted image (**c**). On the diffusion-weighted images (**a, b**), findings include several small lacunar infarcted areas (arrow) of varying age as well as chronic defects (forked arrows). On the T2*-weighted sequence (**c**), the hemosiderin deposits (arrowhead) in the parietooccipital region are most clearly visualized as marked hypointensities.

Differential Diagnosis

Microvascular bleeding due to hypertension	– History of hypertension – Deep structures such as basal ganglia and thalami affected
Ischemic insult with microvascular bleeding	– Multifocal hemosiderin deposits – Hemorrhagic lacunar infarctions
Multiple cavernous malformations	– Usually enhance, popcorn-shaped, usually younger patients
Trauma	– History
Hemorrhagic metastasis	– History of tumor – Contrast enhancement

Tips and Pitfalls

Amyloid angiopathy should be considered in patients with normal blood pressure and a lobar pattern of bleeding.

Selected References

Oide T et al. Relationship between lobar intracerebral hemorrhage and leukoencephalopathy associated with cerebral amyloid angiopathy: clinicopathological study of 64 Japanese patients. Amyloid 2003; 10: 136–143

Thanvi B, Robinson T. Sporadic cerebral amyloid angiopathy—an important cause of cerebral haemorrhage in older people. Age Ageing 2006; 35: 565–571

Yoshimura M et al. Dementia in cerebral amyloid angiopathy: a clinicopathological study. J Neurol 1992; 239: 441–450

Definition

Nontraumatic intracerebral hemorrhage.

▶ **Epidemiology**
Incidence: 12–15 : 100 000 ● Incidence doubles with each decade of life.

▶ **Etiology, pathophysiology, pathogenesis**
Hypertension ● Amyloid angiopathy ● Tumor ● AVM ● Coagulation disorder (iatrogenic, such as coumarin anticoagulant; endogenous, such as leukemia) ● Vasculitis ● Sinus or venous thrombosis ● Aneurysm.

Imaging Signs

▶ **Modality of choice**
CT ● MRI.

▶ **CT findings**
Demarcated hyperdense area ● Halo that becomes increasingly hypodense over time ● Intraventricular, subarachnoid, or subdural component may be present.

▶ **MRI findings**
  – T2 and T2*-weighted images: Hypointense area with susceptibility artifacts.
  – T1-weighted images: Initially hypointense area ● Area becomes hyperintense over time.

▶ **DSA findings**
Usually normal.

Clinical Aspects

▶ **Typical presentation**
Acute neurologic symptoms depending on the location.

▶ **Therapeutic options**
Conservative ● Surgical removal is indicated where there is a significant mass effect.

▶ **Course and prognosis**
Neurologic symptoms usually resolve well ● Risk of recurrent bleeding.

▶ **What does the clinician want to know?**
Extent of the bleeding ● Etiology ● Involvement of crucial areas ● Risk of development of hydrocephalus ● Risk of recurrent bleeding.

Differential Diagnosis

Bleeding from a tumor	– History
	– Location
Vascular malformation	– Flow voids
	– Atypical location
	– Early venous drainage
Amyloid angiopathy	– Usually lobar
	– Patient age

Fig. 1.21 Spontaneous intracerebral hemorrhage. CT. Severe hyperdense hemorrhage with local mass effect. Spread to the ventricular system with intraventricular hemorrhage components.

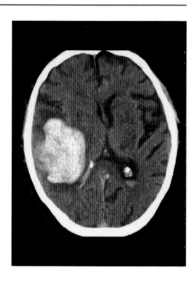

Tips and Pitfalls

Misinterpreting the etiology.

Selected References

Pantazis G et al. Early surgical treatment vs conservative management for spontaneous supratentorial intracerebral hematomas: a prospective randomized study. Surg Neurol 2006; 66: 492–501

Skidmore CT, Andrefsky J. Spontaneous intracerebral hemorrhage: epidemiology, pathophysiology, and medical management. Neurosurg Clin North Am 2002; 13: 281–288

Wu G et al. Spontaneous intracerebral hemorrhage in humans: hematoma enlargement, clot lysis, and brain edema. Acta Neurochir Suppl 2006; 96: 78–80

Definition

▶ **Epidemiology**

Hypertension is the cause of over half of all intracerebral hemorrhages ● 10–15% of all patients with hypertension and spontaneous hemorrhage have an underlying aneurysm or AVM.

▶ **Etiology, pathophysiology, pathogenesis**

Acute: hypertensive crisis ● *Chronic:* degenerative changes in the vascular wall.

– Chronic hypertension leads to degenerative changes in the vascular wall with atherosclerosis and fibrinoid necrosis with or without development of aneurysms ● Sudden pressure peaks cause perforating arteries to rupture, likely from microaneurysms located in the vessel wall ● This explains why lesions usually occur in the basal ganglia.

Imaging Signs

▶ **Modality of choice**

CT ● MRI or MRA where the cause of bleeding is unclear.

▶ **CT findings**

Unenhanced CT shows an ellipsoid or irregularly demarcated hyperdense mass ● Lesion is often located between the putamen and insula in the thalamus, or pons ● May spread to the ventricular system, causing hydrocephalus ● Axial or horizontal herniation can occur.

▶ **MRI findings**

– T2 and T2*-weighted images: Large hypointense area ● Susceptibility artifacts occur over time ● Multifocal hypointense lesion is seen in chronic hypertension.

– T1-weighted images: Hyperintense area ● After contrast administration, enhancement is seen only in hemorrhages from other causes such as AVM or tumors.

▶ **DSA findings**

Almost invariably normal ● Can manifest with mass effect.

Clinical Aspects

▶ **Typical presentation**

Symptoms are indistinguishable from those of an ischemic insult ● Neurologic symptoms depend on the location and extent of hemorrhage ● Loss of consciousness may result ● Symptoms of elevated intracranial pressure (nausea, vomiting, headache) may be present ● Seizures may occur where bleeding is initially lobar.

Fig. 1.22 Hypertensive hemorrhage. CT. Extensive hyperdense demarcated massive hemorrhage originating in the basal ganglia. Severe local edema. Signs of horizontal herniation.

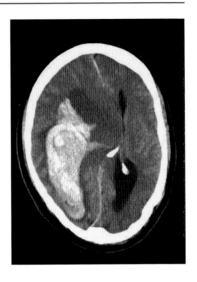

▶ **Therapeutic options**

Conservative ● Ventricular drainage is indicated for intraventricular hemorrhage ● Neurosurgical decompression is indicated when significant mass effect is present.

▶ **Course and prognosis**

Prognosis depends on the location and extend of hemorrhage ● Extensive hemorrhage with ventricular involvement is associated with high mortality ● About 35% of survivors are severely disabled.

▶ **What does the clinician want to know?**

Severity of bleeding ● Ventricular involvement ● Signs of herniation ● Exclude other causes.

Differential Diagnosis

Hemorrhage in the basal ganglia:

Coagulation disorder	– History – Coagulation parameters
Hemorrhagic tumor	– Mixed signal on MRI – Contrast enhancement
Medication or drug misuse	– History – Drug screening

Lobar bleeding:

Amyloid angiopathy	– Older patient – Normal blood pressure – Demented
Thrombosed AVM, dural arteriovenous shunts	– Young patient with typical angiography findings
Thrombosed cortical veins	– MR venography

Small multifocal hemorrhages:

Cavernous or capillary malformation	– Multifocal – Usually minor hemorrhages – Spinal involvement
Amyloid angiopathy	– Older patient – Normal blood pressure – Demented

Tips and Pitfalls

Misinterpreting the cause of bleeding.

Selected References

Ferro JM. Update on intracerebral haemorrhage. J Neurol 2006; 253: 985–999

Huttner HB et al. Influence of intraventricular hemorrhage and occlusive hydrocephalus on the long-term outcome of treated patients with basal ganglia hemorrhage: a case-control study. J Neurosurg 2006; 105: 412–417

Woo D et al. Effect of untreated hypertension on hemorrhagic stroke. Stroke 2004; 35: 1703–1708

Definition

Synonyms: Arteriolosclerosis • Small vessel disease • Microangiopathy • Periventricular leukoencephalopathy • *Severe form:* Binswanger disease, subcortical arteriosclerotic encephalopathy.

▶ **Epidemiology**
Vascular dementia is the third most common form of dementia.

▶ **Etiology, pathophysiology, pathogenesis**
Vessels of intermediate size with a long intraparenchymal course react more sensitively to depressed or elevated blood pressure than do cortical vessels as ambient conditions restrict autoregulation and are less conducive to collateralization.

Imaging Signs

▶ **Modality of choice**
MRI.

▶ **CT findings**
Multiple partially confluent poorly demarcated hypodense areas.

▶ **MRI findings**
– T2-weighted images: Hyperintense areas consisting of small demarcated foci and/or nodular confluent lesions.
– T1-weighted images: Hypointense areas comprising small demarcated foci and/or nodular confluent lesions, but generally less clearly discernable than on T2-weighted images.
– MRA: Extracranial or intracranial stenoses are occasionally demonstrated.

▶ **DSA findings**
Stenoses of smaller and larger vessels.

Clinical Aspects

▶ **Typical presentation**
Common form: Asymptomatic or transient ischemic attack • *Severe form:* Dementia, bulbar paralysis, and/or motor symptoms.

▶ **Therapeutic options**
The common form requires no treatment • Prognosis is good • Aggregation inhibitors • Severe form requires treatment of possible underlying hypertension.

▶ **Course and prognosis**
Course is gradually progressive.

▶ **What does the clinician want to know?**
Extent of white matter damage • Exclude other types of ischemia.

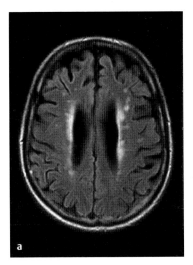
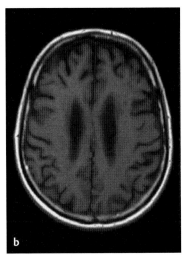

Fig. 1.23 a, b   Ischemia of minor vessels. Axial dark-fluid sequence (**a**) and T1-weighted sequence (**b**). Hyperintense partially nodular, partially confluent lesions on the dark-fluid sequence. Lesions appear hypointense on the T1-weighted sequence.

Differential Diagnosis

Multiple sclerosis

– Often affects younger patients
– Possible spinal cord involvement
– CSF findings

Prominent Virchow–Robin spaces

– Central contrast enhancement

Tips and Pitfalls

Can be misinterpreted as multiple sclerosis.

Selected References

Enzinger C et al. Progression of cerebral white matter lesions—clinical and radiological considerations. J Neurol Sci 2007; 15: 5–10

Guermazi A et al. Neuroradiological findings in vascular dementia. Neuroradiology 2007; 49: 1–22

Matsusue E et al. White matter changes in elderly people: MR-pathologic correlations. Magn Reson Med Sci 2006; 5: 99–104

Definition

▶ **Epidemiology**
Multifactorial systemic disease process • Second most common cause of ischemic insult after thromboembolism from the heart or internal carotid artery.

▶ **Etiology, pathophysiology, pathogenesis**
Degenerative process of the tunica intima • Predisposing factors include hyperlipidemia and cholesteremia • Increasing accumulation of plasma fats, connective tissue fibers, tissue macrophages, and blood components in the vessel wall • Calcifying plaques • Finally ulceration of the intima and thrombus deposition occurs • This leads to progressive narrowing of the lumen • Spread of emboli • Poststenotic dilation • Fusiform aneurysms.

Imaging Signs

▶ **Modality of choice**
MRA • CTA • DSA.

▶ **CT findings**
Lacunar infarcts • Leukoencephalopathy • *CTA:* Irregular narrowing of the lumen with marginal calcifications.

▶ **MRI findings**
– T2-weighted images: reduced fluid signal in the vessels • Medullary hyperintensities consistent with lacunar infarcts and leukoencephalopathy.
– T1-weighted images: normal findings.
– MRA: Stenosis • Ectasia or wall irregularities • *Caution:* Often overestimated.

▶ **DSA findings**
Stenoses • Irregularities of the lumen • Rarely ectasia and elongation of the intracranial arteries.

Clinical Aspects

▶ **Typical presentation**
Stroke or transient ischemic attack (TIA) in the affected arterial territory.

▶ **Therapeutic options**
Diet • Exercise • Aggregation inhibitors and medical reduction of lipid levels • Angioplasty with stent implantation • EC/IC bypass.

▶ **Course and prognosis**
Without aggressive therapy, the disease is progressive with a poor prognosis • Therapy produces only moderate improvement.

▶ **What does the clinician want to know?**
Differential diagnosis • Extent of vascular involvement.

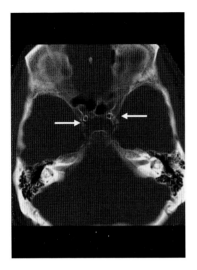

Fig. 1.24 Intracranial atherosclerosis. Unenhanced CT. Bilateral marginal calcifications of the internal carotid arteries (arrows), which are better demarcated in the bone window than in the soft tissue window.

Differential Diagnosis

Vasospasm	– Subarachnoid hemorrhage
Vasculitis and arteritis	– Smaller branches
	– Bleeding often occurs
Moya-moya disease	– Basilar artery is spared
	– "Cloud of smoke"
Dissection	– Intramural hematoma
	– Possible intimal flap

Tips and Pitfalls

Overestimating the stenosis on MRA.

Selected References

Lernfelt B et al. Cerebral atherosclerosis as predictor of stroke and mortality in representative elderly population. Stroke 2002; 33: 224–229

Suwanwela NC, Chutinetr A. Risk factors for atherosclerosis of cervicocerebral arteries: intracranial versus extracranial. Neuroepidemiology 2003; 22: 37–40

Zaidat OO et al. Asymptomatic middle cerebral artery stenosis diagnosed by magnetic resonance angiography. Neuroradiology 2004; 46: 49–53

Brain

Definition

▶ **Epidemiology**
Most common cause of severe disability or death worldwide ● Most common cause of long-term disability.

▶ **Etiology, pathophysiology, pathogenesis**
Embolic occlusion of a cranial artery occurs in three-quarters of cases ● This results in parenchymal damage because of lack of oxygen and nutrients.

Imaging Signs

▶ **Modality of choice**
CT ● MRI.

▶ **CT findings**
Exclude hemorrhage.
- *Early stage:* Dense middle cerebral artery in up to 50% of cases ● Loss of corticomedullary differentiation ● Indistinct lentiform nucleus ● Insula is obliterated ● Gyri are swollen and edematous ● Sulci are narrowed ● Hypodense parenchyma ● Hemorrhagic transformation (24–48 hours) may be visible.
- *Late stage:* Encephalomalacia.
- *CTA:* Occlusion of a main branch in vascular territory.
- *Perfusion CT:* Reduced perfusion of the affected area of the brain (prolonged time to peak).

▶ **MRI findings**
- T2-weighted images: Hyperintense area.
- T1-weighted images: Normal findings in the early phase ● Later, hypointense demarcation of the infarcted area.
- Diffusion-weighted images: Diffusion restriction on B image ● Darkness on ADC map.
- Perfusion-weighted images: 25% of all insults are only positive on perfusion or are larger than on diffusion (mismatch) ● Damage to the ischemic penumbra is still reversible in the acute phase.
- T2*-weighted images: Hypointense cortex after hemorrhagic transformation.

▶ **DSA**
Only where local thrombolysis is indicated.

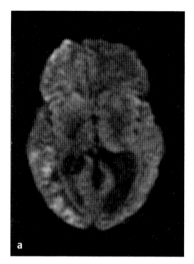 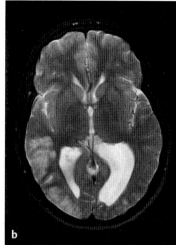

Fig. 1.25 a, b Acute ischemic insult in the right parietooccipital region. Diffusion-weighted sequence (b = 1000) (**a**). Diffusion restriction. T2-weighted image (**b**). Cortical edema in corresponding distribution.

Clinical Aspects

▶ **Typical presentation**
This depends on the affected vessel and the resulting location of the ischemia.

▶ **Therapeutic options**
Systemic intravenous thrombolysis (up to 3 hours) ● Local intraarterial thrombolysis (3–6 hours in the anterior vascular system, > 3 hours in the vertebrobasilar vascular system) ● Mechanical thrombectomy where indicated ● Angioplasty with or without placement of a stent ● Heparinization may be indicated after more than 6 hours ● Rehabilitation measures ● Reduction of risk factors ● Medical aggregation inhibition.

▶ **Course and prognosis**
Depends on the extent and location of the ischemic insult and on the patient's age.

▶ **What does the clinician want to know?**
Exclude intracranial hemorrhage ● Age of the ischemic insult ● Extent of the reversibly and irreversibly damaged areas.

Differential Diagnosis

Other diagnoses involving the dense middle cerebral artery sign
– Atherosclerosis (compare with contralateral side)
– High hematocrit, dehydration
– Relative increase in vascular density against a hypodense parenchyma

Tips and Pitfalls

Overlooking the early signs of ischemic insult.

Selected References

Adams HP et al. Guidelines for the early management of patients with ischemic stroke: a scientific statement from the Stroke Council of the American Stroke Association. Stroke 2003; 34: 1056–1083

Fiebach JB et al. Stroke magnetic resonance imaging is accurate in hyperacute intracerebral hemorrhage: a multicenter study on the validity of stroke imaging. Stroke 2004; 35: 502–506

von Kummer R et al. Acute stroke: Usefulness of early CT findings before thrombolytic therapy. Radiology 1997; 205: 327–333

Sunshine JL. CT, MR imaging, and MR angiography in the evaluation of patients with acute stroke. J Vasc Interv Radiol 2004; 15: 47–55

Definition

Round dilation of the vascular wall ● Usually at vascular bifurcations ● 70–75% are solitary, 25–30% are multiple.

▶ **Epidemiology**

Present at autopsy in 0.4–10% (with ethnic variation) ● 85% occur in the anterior vascular system and only 15% in the posterior vascular system ● 30–35% occur in the anterior communicating artery ● 30–35% in the posterior communicating artery ● 20% in the middle cerebral artery ● 15% in the vertebrobasilar system.

▶ **Etiology, pathophysiology, pathogenesis**

Aneurysms usually occur due to vascular injury from hemodynamic causes in the setting of atherosclerosis, less often due to trauma or infection.

- *Risk factors:* High blood pressure ● Certain anatomic variants of the circle of Willis ● Smoking ● Alcohol abuse ● Anticoagulation medication ● Oral contraceptives.
- Increased risk of rupture exists especially with sudden and intense increase in blood pressure ● Increased familial incidence and hereditary predisposition in Ehlers–Danlos syndrome type IV, neurofibromatosis type I, fibromuscular dysplasia, and autosomal dominant kidney degeneration.

Imaging Signs

▶ **Modality of choice**

CTA ● MRI ● DSA.

▶ **CT findings**

Often normal ● CTA is very sensitive in searching for aneurysms.

▶ **MRI findings**

- T2-weighted images: Round area with a flow signal, adjacent to one of the proximal cerebral arteries.
- T1-weighted images: Normal ● Occasionally a round enhancing structure will be visualized.
- MRA: Sensitive in searching for aneurysms ● Aneurysm size is often underestimated.

▶ **DSA findings**

Provides the most reliable information about size, configuration (lobulated/not lobulated), width of the neck of the aneurysm, relationship to and course of vessels ● Can demonstrate other smaller aneurysms ● 3D rotational angiography provides precise information about vascular structures ● DSA may be combined with endovascular therapy ● Purely diagnostic DSA is not indicated where CTA and/or MRI are available.

Clinical Aspects

▶ **Typical presentation**

Clinical findings are normal (incidental finding) ● Rupture produces an extensive subarachnoid hemorrhage, occasionally with a "thunderclap" headache or initial

Fig. 1.26 a–c Saccular aneurysm (arrows). Aneurysm of the anterior communicating artery (**a, b**). 3D reconstruction of CTA (**a**), 3D reconstruction of DSA (**b**). Aneurysm of the posterior cerebral artery (MRA) (**c**).

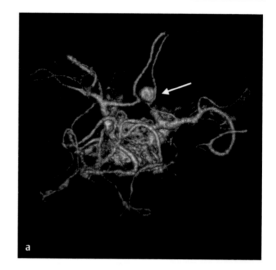

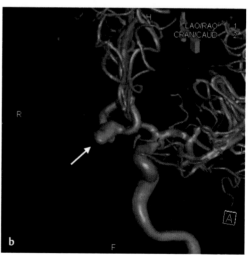

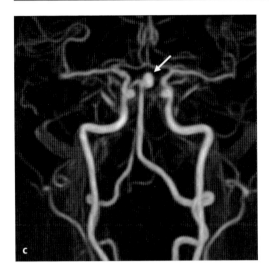

loss of consciousness ● Vegetative symptoms (sweating; vomiting; rise or drop in blood pressure; fluctuations in temperature, pulse, and respiration) ● Patient may be disoriented ● Meningism may be present ● Rarely there will be a focal neurologic deficit.

▶ **Therapeutic options**
Endovascular occlusion with platinum coils (method of choice in acute subarachnoid hemorrhage and elective) ● Follow-up examinations at regularly intervals are indicated for incidental findings of smaller aneurysms (< 5 mm, not lobulated) until they reach the size where intervention is indicated ● Risk factors should be reduced (quit smoking, stabilize blood pressure, discontinue platelet aggregation inhibitors) ● Where indicated in acute cases, massive hemorrhage is drained and aneurysm managed by neurosurgical clipping or wrapping ● Elective clipping or wrapping.

▶ **Course and prognosis**
Mortality before reaching the hospital is 35% ● 25% mortality in the hospital ● 50% of survivors have permanent damage ● Prognosis depends on the extent of the subarachnoid hemorrhage, the clinical sequelae (Hunt and Huss classification), and possible complications, such as vasospasm and hydrocephalus ● The aneurysm may reoccur after treatment.

▶ **What does the clinician want to know?**
Size ● Width of the neck ● Shape ● Indication for intervention.

Differential Diagnosis

Vascular sling	– Multiple views – 3D rotational angiography may be indicated
Subarachnoid hemorrhage from other causes (traumatic or idiopathic)	– History – CTA, MRA to exclude aneurysm
Perimesencephalic bleeding without evidence of an aneurysm	– In 10% of all subarachnoid hemorrhages – Pay attention to venous phase on DSA
Cocaine misuse	– History – Drug screening
Cranial AVM	– Early venous drainage

Tips and Pitfalls

Misinterpreting aneurysm as a vascular sling • Aneurysm can be missed on certain projections.

Selected References

Adams WM et al. The role of MR angiography in the pretreatment assessment of intracranial aneurysms: A comparative study. AJNR Am J Neuroradiol 2000; 21: 1618–1628

Johnston SC et al. Endovascular and surgical treatment of unruptured cerebral aneurysms: Comparison of risks. Ann Neurol 2000; 48: 11–19

Wiebers DO, International Study of Unruptured Intracranial Aneurysms Investigators. Unruptured intracranial aneurysms: Natural history, clinical outcome, and risks of surgical and endovascular treatment. Lancet 2003; 362: 103–110

Yong-Zhong G, van Alphen HA. Pathogenesis and histopathology of saccular aneurysms: Review of the literature. Neurol Res 1990; 12: 249–255

Definition

No synonym.

Aneurysm with a maximum diameter exceeding 25 mm.

▶ **Epidemiology**
Accounts for 5–8% of all aneurysms.

▶ **Etiology, pathophysiology, pathogenesis**
Sixty percent occur in the internal carotid artery (usually in the cavernous segment) ● 40% are calcified.

Imaging Signs

▶ **Modality of choice**
DSA.

▶ **CT findings**
Large round structure ● Marked homogeneous enhancement ● Calcification is readily visible where present.

▶ **MRI findings**
– T2-weighted images: Large round structure with flow void ● Hyperintense edematous zone is often present in the surrounding brain parenchyma.
– T1-weighted images: Round structure with flow void ● Often there will be a hyperintense marginal signal from thrombi.
– T1-weighted contrast images: Marked enhancement ● Thrombi do not enhance.
– MRA: Turbulent flows often cause the lesion to appear too small ● Hypointense especially on the time-of-flight sequences.

▶ **DSA findings**
Visualizes giant aneurysm in relation to the underlying vessel.

Clinical Aspects

▶ **Typical presentation**
Occurs only in 25–35% of all subarachnoid hemorrhages ● Symptoms usually include a mass effect (75% of all lesions), intracerebral hemorrhage, or stroke due to the disseminated thrombi arising in the aneurysm ● Headache.

▶ **Therapeutic options**
Clipping and/or coiling is often difficult ● Recanalization often occurs after coiling ● Occlusion of the underlying vessel with balloons or coils.

▶ **Course and prognosis**
Unfavorable due to the difficult therapy ● Recanalization often occurs ● Local mass effect.

▶ **What does the clinician want to know?**
Exclude other changes ● Therapeutic options.

Fig. 1.27 a–c Giant aneurysm. Unenhanced CT (**a**) visualizes an extensive, slightly hyperdense giant aneurysm of the left middle cerebral artery. The P-A DSA (**b**) shows partial filling of the aneurysm in the early arterial phase.

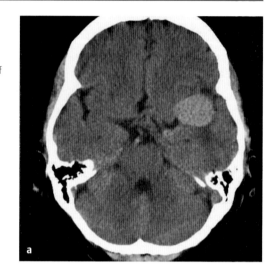

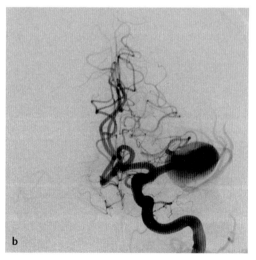

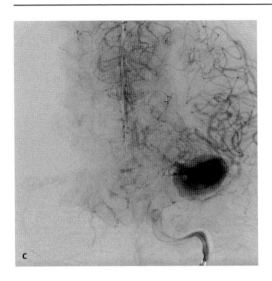

In the late arterial phase of DSA (**c**) the contrast agent remains in the aneurysm with only gradual washout.

Differential Diagnosis

Meningioma	– "Dural tail" sign
	– Blush on DSA
Schwannoma	– Arises from a nerve
Fusiform aneurysm	– Broad-based
	– Usually no calcifications
	– No mass effect

Tips and Pitfalls

Can be misinterpreted as a meningioma, schwannoma, or fusiform aneurysm.

Selected References

Blanc R et al. Delayed stroke secondary to increasing mass effect after endovascular treatment of a giant aneurysm by parent vessel occlusion. AJNR Am J Neuroradiol 2001; 22: 1841–1843

Definition

Dilated, tortuous, and elongated vessel ● Dolichoectasia ● No aneurysm neck.

▶ **Epidemiology**
Most common locations: Distal vertebral artery ● Basilar artery ● P1 segment of the posterior cerebral artery ● Supraclinoid (cerebral) segment of the internal carotid artery.

▶ **Etiology, pathophysiology, pathogenesis**
The most common cause is atherosclerosis ● Rare causes include immunosuppression (HIV), viruses (varicella), or collagen diseases.

Imaging Signs

▶ **Modality of choice**
DSA.

▶ **CT findings**
Ectatic artery ● Marginal calcifications.

▶ **MRI findings**
T2-weighted images show an ectatic artery with a flow void ● MRA shows a turbulent flow ● Best visualized on T1-weighted sequences with contrast.

▶ **DSA findings**
Focal aneurysmal ectasia of an artery ● No evidence of an aneurysm neck.

Clinical Aspects

▶ **Typical presentation**
Usually transient ischemic attack or stroke ● Less often subarachnoid hemorrhage.

▶ **Therapeutic options**
Endovascular therapy is usually difficult in the absence of an aneurysm neck ● Stent placement for remodeling may be indicated ● In selected cases, occlusion of the entire artery may be attempted ● Neurosurgical therapy is occasionally indicated.

▶ **Course and prognosis**
Usually progressive worsening occurs, leading to severe disabilities or death.

▶ **What does the clinician want to know?**
Differentiate from treatable aneurysms ● Extent of the damage to the affected vessel ● Mass effect on structures such as the brainstem.

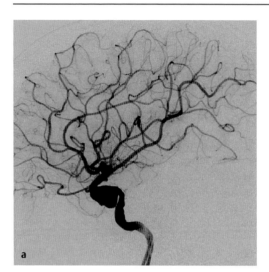

Fig. 1.28 a, b Fusiform aneurysm. Lateral (**a**) and P-A DSA (**b**). Fusiform aneurysm in the cavernous segment of the internal carotid artery.

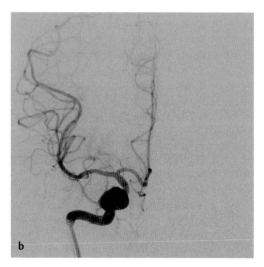

Differential Diagnosis

Vertebrobasilar artery dolichoectasia	– Pseudoaneurysm
	– Tends to be ectatic
Giant Aneurysm	– An aneurysm neck is usually demonstrated

Tips and Pitfalls

Can be misinterpreted as vertebrobasilar artery dolichoectasia or giant aneurysm.

Selected References

Drake CG, Peerless SJ. Giant fusiform intracranial aneurysms: Review of 120 patients treated surgically from 1965 to 1992. J Neurosurg 1997; 87: 141–162

Definition

A better term would be "infectious aneurysm" • The aneurysm is "bacterial" or "mycotic" only where bacteria or fungi are the cause.

▶ **Epidemiology**
Accounts for 2–3% of all aneurysms.

▶ **Etiology, pathophysiology, pathogenesis**
Septic embolus • Leukocyte infiltration into the vascular wall as far as the tunica media • Usually in the Virchow–Robin spaces with secondary weakening of the vascular wall • Usually occurs at multiple locations in the distal branches of the middle cerebral artery • Aneurysm develops within 24 hours of a septic embolus • Pathogens usually spread from heart valves colonized by streptococcus in endocarditis • Fungi are rarely the cause; fungal cause is usually found with craniofacial infection • In fungal infections, the aneurysm usually develops over the course of several months.

Imaging Signs

▶ **Modality of choice**
DSA.

▶ **CT findings**
Subarachnoid hemorrhage may be demonstrated • Occasionally there will be a round enhancement along distal arteries.

▶ **MRI**
  – T2-weighted images: Small round structure with flow void in the subarachnoid space.
  – T1-weighted images: Small round enhancement along distal arteries.

▶ **DSA findings**
A small aneurysm is visualized along distal branches of the arteries supplying the brain.

Clinical Aspects

▶ **Typical presentation**
Subarachnoid hemorrhage with headache.

▶ **Therapeutic options**
Antibiotic or antimycotic medication • Endovascular or neurosurgical treatment is contraindicated due to the high risk of rupture • Surgical decompression may be required in the presence of extensive subarachnoid hemorrhage with mass effect.

▶ **Course and prognosis**
Regress or disappear under antibiotic therapy • Rupture leads to extensive subarachnoid hemorrhage.

▶ **What does the clinician want to know?**
Rule out noninfectious aneurysms or other changes.

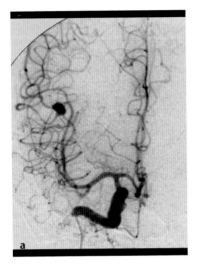 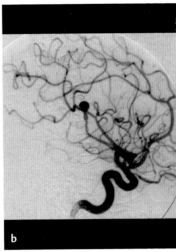

Fig. 1.29 a, b Mycotic aneurysm. P-A (**a**) and lateral (**b**) DSA. Typical distal location of a mycotic aneurysm along a branch of the middle cerebral artery.

Differential Diagnosis

Saccular aneurysm	– Tends to occur along proximal segments of the vessel
Meningioma	– "Dural tail" sign – Marked enhancement
Glioma	– Not in the subarachnoid space – No contrast filling on DSA

Tips and Pitfalls

Missing the aneurysm ● Endovascular therapy.

Selected References

Barrow DL, Prats AR. Infectious intracranial aneurysms: Comparison of groups with and without endocarditis. Neurosurgery 1990; 27: 562–572

Brust JC et al. The diagnosis and treatment of cerebral mycotic aneurysms. Ann Neurol 1990; 27: 238–246

Definition

▶ **Epidemiology**
  Accounts for 1% of all acute insults.
▶ **Etiology, pathophysiology, pathogenesis**
  Infectious and septic as in otitis media • Bland thromboses such as those from exogenous hormones, in hematologic disorders, postpartum, or posttraumatic • Occasionally idiopathic.

Imaging Signs

▶ **Modality of choice**
  MRV.
▶ **CT findings**
  Used to exclude hemorrhage • Diffuse or focal cerebral edema • Hyperdense sinus • Hemorrhagic infarcts • Local hyperemia • Contrast filling defects ("empty triangle" sign) • Collateral veins.
▶ **MRV findings**
  Signal depends on the age of the thrombus • Directly visualizes thrombosed veins in the brain • Typical "empty triangle" sign is seen in acute thrombi in the confluence of the sinuses.
▶ **DSA**
  Indicated only where previous studies are inconclusive.

Clinical Aspects

▶ **Typical presentation**
  Can be asymptomatic • Symptoms depend on the location and extent of the impairment to venous drainage • Signs of elevated intracranial pressure (headache, nausea, vomiting, impaired vigilance) • Focal signs include unilateral cerebral symptoms and focal seizures • Coma or death may occur.
▶ **Therapeutic options**
  Systemic administration of heparin • Exceptional cases may require endovascular thrombolysis.
▶ **Course and prognosis**
  A hemorrhagic infarction develops in half of all cases.
▶ **What does the clinician want to know?**
  Exclude other causes.

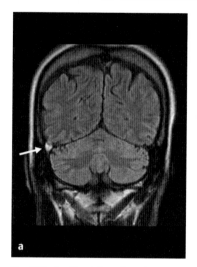 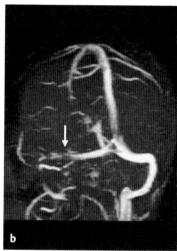

Fig. 1.30 a, b Dural sinus thrombosis. MR image, coronal dark-fluid sequence (**a**). The transverse sinus (arrow) is occluded by thrombosis and appears hyperintense. Venous time-of-flight MRA (**b**). Right transverse sinus ends abruptly (arrow).

Differential Diagnosis

Hypoplastic or aplastic transverse sinus as a congenital anatomic variant

– Comparison with coronal and axial slices

Pacchioni (arachnoid) granulations simulating a filling defect

– Proximal and distal sinus are normal

Tips and Pitfalls

Because this is often overlooked, a meticulous diagnostic workup is required.

Selected References

Ayanzen RH et al. Cerebral MR venography: normal anatomy and potential diagnostic pitfalls. AJNR Am J Neuroradiol 2000; 21: 74–78

Ferro JM et al. Interobserver agreement in the magnetic resonance location of cerebral vein and dural sinus thrombosis. Eur J Neurol 2007; 14: 353–356

Khandelwal N et al. Comparison of CT venography with MR venography in cerebral sinovenous thrombosis. AJR Am J Roentgenol 2006; 187: 1637–1643

Definition

Occlusion of the aneurysm by a clip or platinum coils • Follow-up examination to evaluate the success of therapy • Used to exclude recurrence of the aneurysm or development of new aneurysms at other locations.

Imaging Signs

▶ **Modality of choice**
  DSA (gold standard).
▶ **CT or CTA findings**
  Metal artifact obscures image.
▶ **MRI findings**
  Caution: Ferromagnetic aneurysm clips interfere with the examination • Coils can cause warming.
  – T2-weighted images: Flow void in the recanalized aneurysm.
  – T1-weighted images: Normal • The recanalized aneurysm may enhance.
  – MRA: Detects recanalization or a new aneurysm > 3 mm.
▶ **DSA findings**
  Detects recanalization or a new aneurysm.

Clinical Aspects

▶ **Typical presentation**
  Postoperative or postinterventional • After subarachnoid hemorrhage or elective procedure.
▶ **Therapeutic options**
  Second intervention.
▶ **Course and prognosis**
  Subarachnoid hemorrhage may reoccur after recanalization or development of a new aneurysm • Rate of retreatment after primary subarachnoid hemorrhage has in some series been reported up to 17% after coiling and 4% after clipping.
▶ **What does the clinician want to know?**
  Recanalization • New aneurysm.

Differential Diagnosis

Thrombosed aneurysm	– Thrombotic material that simulates recanalization on MRI
	– Recanalization masked by metal artifacts on CT or MRI

Tips and Pitfalls

Missing recanalization or a new aneurysm on imaging studies • Recanalization masked by metal artifacts on CT or MRI.

Fig. 1.31 a–d Postcoiling status of an aneurysm of the internal carotid artery. DSA (**a**). Compacted platinum coils (arrow) and partially recanalized aneurysm (forked arrow). Axial MIP view of a time-of-flight sequence (**b**). Platinum coils and recanalization (arrow) are barely distinguishable.

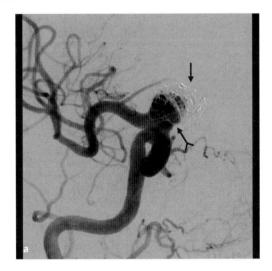

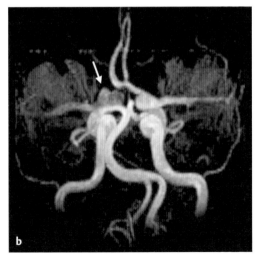

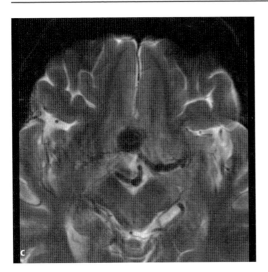

MR axial T2-weighted image (**c**). The entire aneurysm is hypointense. The portion filled by platinum coils and the recanalized portion cannot be clearly differentiated. Source image of the time-of-flight sequence (**d**). The recanalized portion (forked arrow) and the hypointense portion filled by platinum coils (arrow) are distinguishable.

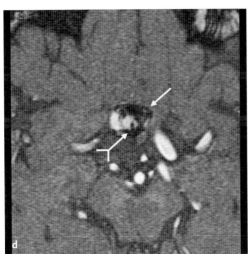

Selected References

Campi A et al. Retreatment of ruptured cerebral aneurysms in patients randomized by coiling or clipping in the International Subarachnoid Aneurysm Trial (ISAT). Stroke 2007; 38: 1538–1544

Cloft HJ et al. Observer agreement in the assessment of endovascular aneurysm therapy and aneurysm recurrence. AJNR Am J Neuroradiol 2007; 28: 497–500

Grunwald IQ et al. Recanalization after endovascular treatment of intracerebral aneurysms. Neuroradiology 2007; 49: 41–47

van der Schaaf IC et al. Multislice computed tomography angiography screening for new aneurysms in patients with previously clip-treated intracranial aneurysms: Feasibility, positive predictive value, and interobserver agreement. J Neurosurg 2006; 105: 682–688

Definition

Surgical anastomosis between a branch of the external carotid artery (typically the superficial temporal artery) and a branch of the internal carotid artery (typically the middle cerebral artery) • *Indication:* Occlusion of the internal carotid artery or middle cerebral artery.

Imaging Signs

▶ **Modality of choice**
MRA or CTA.
▶ **Color-coded duplex sonography**
Good noninvasive modality for follow-up examination.
▶ **CT findings**
Small temporal craniotomy.
▶ **CTA findings**
Visualizes the bypass • Sensitivity depends on flow.
▶ **MRI findings**
May detect a flow signal through the craniotomy.
▶ **DSA findings**
Visualizes the bypass with the highest sensitivity.

Clinical Aspects

▶ **Typical presentation**
Postoperative follow-up examination.
▶ **Therapeutic options**
Second intervention.
▶ **Course and prognosis**
This depends on the underlying disorder (i.e., occlusion of the carotid artery or middle cerebral artery).
▶ **What does the clinician want to know?**
Patency of the bypass • Sufficiency of tissue perfusion • Infarcts.

Tips and Pitfalls

Misinterpreting flow phenomena along the craniotomy • Misinterpreting delayed filling of the middle cerebral artery flow tract as insufficiency of the EC/IC bypass.

Selected References

Horn P et al. Evaluation of extracranial-intracranial arterial bypass function with magnetic resonance angiography. Neuroradiology 2004; 46: 723–729

McDowell F, Flamm ES. EC/IC bypass study. Stroke 1986; 17: 1–2

Fig. 1.32 EC/IC bypass. DSA in coronal projection. The middle cerebral artery flow tract is filled via the external carotid artery. Incidental findings include a coiled aneurysm of the internal carotid artery (asterisk).

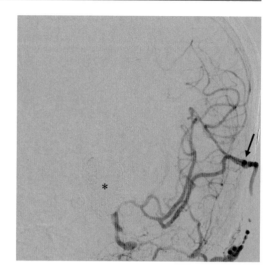

Fig. 1.33 MRA. Right EC/IC bypass (arrow).

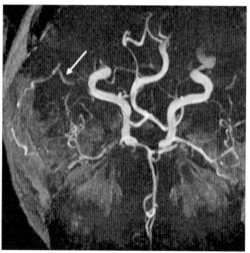

Definition

▶ **Epidemiology**
Manifests itself between the ages of 10 and 30 years.

▶ **Etiology, pathophysiology, pathogenesis**
Anastomoses between arteries and veins of the spinal cord • A nidus and/or direct arteriovenous fistula may be present • Superficial AVMs are only supplied by the pial arteries • Deep AVMs receive their supply from the anterior or posterior spinal artery • Severity can vary from micro-AVMs to large high-flow AVMs • Multiple AVMs can occur • Stenosis or aneurysms of the arterial feeders and ectasias or stenosis of the draining veins can also occur.

Imaging Signs

▶ **Modality of choice**
MRI.

▶ **Contrast CT findings**
Tortuous hyperdensities consistent with blood vessels.

▶ **MRI findings**
– T2-weighted images: Hypointense tortuous flow voids • Hyperintense elongated areas in the spinal cord.
– T1-weighted images: Normal • Tortuous dilated vessels are visible after contrast administration.

▶ **DSA**
Spinal angiography visualizes vascular architecture and blood flow with greater precision and is useful for planning treatment • DSA in combination with endovascular therapy is recommended.

Clinical Aspects

▶ **Typical presentation**
Hemodynamic dysfunction due to an arterial steal effect (ischemia) or due to venous stasis • Paresis • Hemorrhage • Lumbago or radicular pain • Sensory changes • Impotence • Bladder and rectal disorders.

▶ **Therapeutic options**
Embolization • Surgery • Radiation therapy is rarely indicated.

▶ **Course and prognosis**
Myelomalacia • Edema • Spinal cord atrophy • Untreated cases have a poor long-term prognosis.

▶ **What does the clinician want to know?**
Diagnosis • Exclude spinal dural arteriovenous fistula • Location of the arterial feeder • Embolization where indicated.

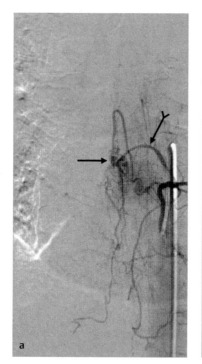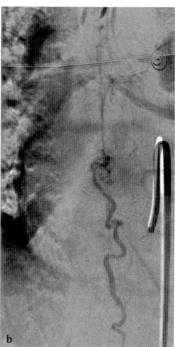

Fig. 2.1a, b   Spinal arteriovenous malformation. DSA. The malformation (arrow) is supplied by a radicular arterial branch (**a**, forked arrow) and drains into an ectatic spinal vein (**b**).

Differential Diagnosis

Intramedullary tumor, astrocytoma	– No vascular dilation
	– Contrast enhancement
	– Multisegmental
Ependymoma	– Marked enhancement
	– Diffuse growth
Cavernous hemangioma	– No vascular dilation

Tips and Pitfalls

Cases with a slowly progressive clinical course may be diagnosed late.

Selected References

Mascalchi M et al. MR angiography of spinal vascular malformations. AJNR Am J Neuroradiol 1995; 16: 289–297

Strom RG et al. Frequency of spinal arteriovenous malformations in patients with unexplained myelopathy. Neurology 2006; 66: 928–931

Thron A et al. [Spinal arteriovenous malformations.] Radiologe 2001; 41: 949–954 [In German]

Definition

▶ **Epidemiology**
Manifests itself between the ages of 50 and 70 years • 85% of patients are men.

▶ **Etiology, pathophysiology, pathogenesis**
Anastomosis between meningeal arteries and intradural veins • Spinal hypoxia occurs due to elevated intraspinal pressure • Usually occurs at the level of the middle thoracic spine or at the thoracolumbar junction.

Imaging Signs

▶ **Modality of choice**
MRI • DSA.

▶ **CT findings**
The affected segment, usually the distal spinal cord, is distended • Enhancing dilated veins are visualized on the surface of the spinal cord.

▶ **MRI findings**
  – T2-weighted images: Hyperintense, swollen spinal cord • Hypointense, tortuous vessels • Hyperintense CSF around the vessels.
  – T1-weighted images: Dilated vessels and spinal cord enhance with contrast.

▶ **DSA**
Precisely visualizes vascular architecture and blood flow.

Clinical Aspects

▶ **Typical presentation**
Slowly progressive sensorimotor myelopathy • Paresis • Sensory changes • Back or radicular pain • Impotence • Bladder and rectal disorders.

▶ **Therapeutic options**
Endovascular or surgical obliteration of the fistula.

▶ **Course and prognosis**
With prompt therapy, neurologic symptoms may be reversible • Untreated cases exhibit a slowly progressive clinical course • The final outcome is paraplegia.

▶ **What does the clinician want to know?**
Extent of spinal cord damage • Extent of thrombosis • Evaluation of the adjacent segments of the arterial feeders and draining veins • Etiology of the thrombosis • Acute or previous pulmonary embolism.

Differential Diagnosis

Dural AVM	– Hemorrhage is common
Amyotrophic lateral sclerosis	– Clinically distinguishable

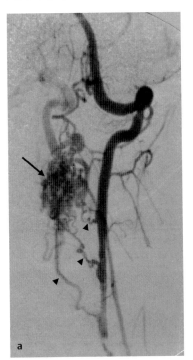
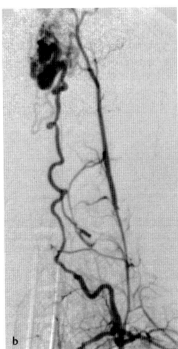

Fig. 2.2 a, b Spinal dural arteriovenous fistula. DSA. The fistula (arrow) is supplied by meningeal branches (arrowheads) of the vertebral artery (**a**) and ascending cervical artery (**b**).

Tips and Pitfalls

Due to its clinical course, it can be misinterpreted as multiple sclerosis or spinal stenosis.

Selected References

Blehaut V et al. Spinal dural arteriovenous fistula with peri-medullary venous drainage: analysis of a series from a single centre and review of the literature. Rev Neurol (Paris) 2006; 162: 1091–1108

Bowen BC et al. Spinal dural arteriovenous fistulas: evaluation with MR angiography. AJNR Am J Neuroradiol 1995; 16: 2029–2043

Koch C et al. [Spinal dural arteriovenous fistula: clinical and radiological finding in 54 patients.] Fortschr Röngenstr 2003; 175: 1071–1078 [In German]

Thron A. [Spinal dural arteriovenous fistulas.] Radiologe 2001; 41: 955–960 [In German]

Definition

▶ **Epidemiology**
Rare anomaly ● Occurs in 1% of the population.

▶ **Etiology, pathophysiology, pathogenesis**
Aplasia of the cervical segment of the internal carotid artery ● The ascending pharyngeal and caroticotympanic arteries act as substitutes ● As a result the internal carotid artery courses through the middle ear.

Imaging Signs

▶ **Modality of choice**
Often an incidental finding ● CT is the modality of choice for this specific line of inquiry.

▶ **CT findings**
Soft tissue structure in the hypotympanum ● Vertical segment of the carotid canal is absent ● Tympanic canaliculus is widened ● There is a defect in the bony plate between the middle ear cavity and the horizontal segment of the carotid canal.

▶ **MRA and DSA findings**
The ectopic vessel narrows where it enters the skull base ● It lies farther lateral and posterior in the petrous bone than normal.

Clinical Aspects

▶ **Typical presentation**
Often asymptomatic ● Pulsatile tinnitus ● Partial hearing loss ● Pain in the ear ● Sensation of fullness in the ear ● Otoscopy reveals redness indistinctly visible through the tympanic membrane.

▶ **Therapeutic options**
None.

▶ **Course and prognosis**
Good.

▶ **What does the clinician want to know?**
Where surgery is planned, the ear surgeon should be aware of the ectopic vessel coursing through the surgical field.

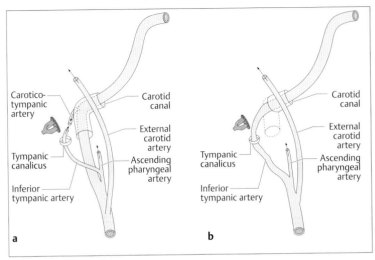

Fig. 3.1 a, b Physiologic (**a**) and ectopic (**b**) course of the internal carotid artery (adapted from Lo et al.).

a Normally, the petrous part of the internal carotid artery consists of a vertical and a horizontal segment. The inferior tympanic artery arising from the ascending pharyngeal artery courses through the tympanic canaliculus to form an anastomosis on the promontory with the caroticotympanic artery, which courses through the caroticotympanic canaliculus.

b In aplasia of the cervical segment of the internal carotid artery, the expanded inferior tympanic and caroticotympanic arteries act as replacements for the internal carotid artery. The vertical segment of the carotid canal is also absent.

Differential Diagnosis

Dehiscence of the jugular bulb	– Jugular bulb protrudes into the middle ear – Jugular fossa is enlarged – Defect in the floor of the hypotympanum
Glomus tympanicum tumor	– Focal mass of soft tissue density in the middle ear cavity
Glomus jugulare tumor	– Widening and erosion of the jugular fossa and occasionally petrous bone as well
Cholesterol granuloma	– Mass of soft tissue density with destruction of the surrounding bone structures – Typically shows high signal intensity on T1-weighted images

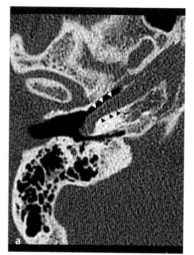
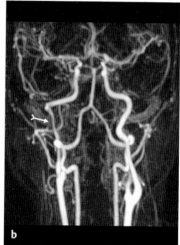

Fig. 3.2 a–c   Aberrant internal carotid artery. Unenhanced CT scan (bone window), axial (**a**), MIP from contrast MRA (**b**), and DSA (**c**). The horizontal segment (triangles) of the ectopic right internal carotid artery bulges into the middle ear without any cortical covering (**a**). The vertical segment (forked arrow) is narrower than on the contralateral side (**b,c**) because the ectopic vessel enters the petrous bone through the tympanic canaliculus.

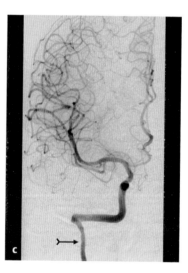

Tips and Pitfalls

Confusing this anomaly with a glomus tumor or another middle ear tumor can have devastating consequences.

Selected References

Botma M et al. Aberrant internal carotid artery in the middle-ear space. J Laryngol Otol 2000; 114: 784–787

Lo WWM et al. Aberrant carotid artery: radiologic diagnosis with emphasis on high-resolution computed tomography. RadioGraphics 1985; 5: 985–993

Sauvaget E et al. Aberrant internal carotid artery in the temporal bone. Arch Otolaryngol Head Neck Surg 2006; 132: 86–91

Definition

▶ **Epidemiology**
Most common vascular anomaly in the petrous bone • Occurs in 3.5–33.5% of the population • Occurs equally often in males and females.

▶ **Etiology, pathophysiology, pathogenesis**
The jugular bulb lies superior to the tympanic ring • Predilection for the right side • Significance of weak or absent mastoid pneumatization is controversial.

Imaging Signs

▶ **Modality of choice**
Incidental finding.

▶ **CT findings**
Round structure with a cortical margin in the posterior petrous bone.

▶ **MRI findings**
Round, markedly enhancing formation in the posterior petrous bone • MR venography confirms the high jugular bulb.

Clinical Aspects

▶ **Typical presentation**
Asymptomatic.

▶ **Therapeutic options**
None.

▶ **Course and prognosis**
Does not increase in size.

▶ **What does the clinician want to know?**
Location of the high jugular bulb relative to masses in the cerebellopontine angle or to the surgical approach.

Differential Diagnosis

Glomus jugulare tumor	– Widening and erosion of the jugular fossa and petrous bone as well in larger tumors – "Salt and pepper" appearance on noncontrast MRI
Schwannoma of the jugular fossa	– Smooth widening of the jugular fossa due to an enhancing tumor but without the "salt and pepper" pattern

Tips and Pitfalls

Can be misinterpreted as a tumor in the jugular fossa or as osteolysis.

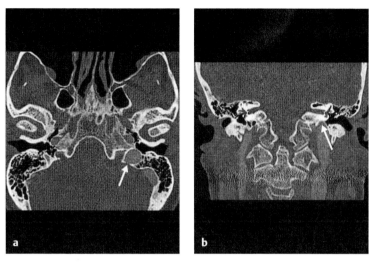

Fig. 3.3 a, b   High jugular bulb. Unenhanced CT (bone window), axial source image (**a**) and coronal reconstruction (**b**). The left jugular bulb (arrow) is covered by a thin layer of bone and projects into the hypotympanum.

Selected References

Atilla S et al. Computed tomographic evaluation of surgically significant vascular variations related to the temporal bone. Eur J Radiol 1995; 20: 52–56

Koesling S et al. Vascular anomalies, sutures and small canals of the temporal bone on axial CT. Eur J Radiol 2005; 54: 335–343

Definition

▶ **Epidemiology**
Occurs in 2.4–7% of the population.
▶ **Etiology, pathophysiology, pathogenesis**
Vascular malformation characterized by a high jugular bulb with dehiscence of the bony mantle.

Imaging Signs

▶ **Modality of choice**
CT or MRI.
▶ **CT findings**
Soft tissue protrudes into the middle ear without bony coverage.
▶ **MRI findings**
On contrast images, the contour of the bulb appears lobulated or drawn out in a long line ● MR venography shows the bulb extending laterally and superiorly into the middle ear spaces.

Clinical Aspects

▶ **Typical presentation**
Often asymptomatic ● Pulsatile tinnitus ● Hearing loss because of impaired sound transmission ● Otoscopy reveals a round bluish mass in the lower third of the tympanum, indistinctly visible through the tympanic membrane.
▶ **Therapeutic options**
None.
▶ **Course and prognosis**
Good.
▶ **What does the clinician want to know?**
The anomaly is a possible risk in any middle ear surgery.

Differential Diagnosis

Ectopic internal carotid artery	– Mass of soft tissue density in the middle ear
	– Vertical segment of the carotid canal is absent
	– Defect in the horizontal segment of the carotid canal
Glomus jugulare tumor	– Widening and erosion of the jugular fossa
	– Widening of the petrous bone as well in larger tumors
	– "Salt and pepper" appearance on noncontrast MRI
Schwannoma of the jugular fossa	– Smooth widening of the jugular fossa

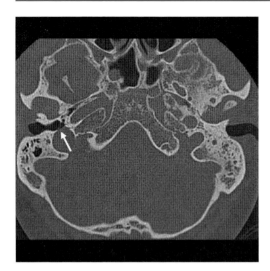

Fig. 3.4 Dehiscence of the jugular bulb (arrow). Transverse unenhanced CT scan (bone window). The right jugular bulb projects into the middle ear without any bony covering (courtesy of Dr. R. Klingebiel, Berlin).

Tips and Pitfalls

Can be confused with a glomus jugulare tumor.

Selected References

Atilla S et al. Computed tomographic evaluation of surgically significant vascular variations related to the temporal bone. Eur J Radiol 1995; 20: 52–56

Hourani R et al. Dehiscence of the jugular bulb and vestibular aqueduct. J Comput Assist Tomogr 2005; 29: 657–662

Tomura N et al. Normal variations of the temporal bone on high-resolution CT: their incidence and clinical significance. Clin Radiol 1995; 50: 144–148

Definition

▶ **Epidemiology**
Rare type of glomus tumor ● Most common primary tumor of the middle ear.

▶ **Etiology, pathophysiology, pathogenesis**
Tumor is usually limited to the middle ear cavity ● Arises from the tympanic plexus of the promontory.

Imaging Signs

▶ **Modality of choice**
CT ● MRI.

▶ **CT findings**
Formation of soft tissue density in the middle ear cavity ● The ossicles of the middle ear are usually intact ● Rarely extends posteriorly into the mastoid or anteriorly into the eustachian tube and nasopharynx.

▶ **MRI findings**
Classic signal behavior ● Hypointense or isointense to muscle on T1-weighted images ● Hyperintense on T2-weighted images ● "Salt and pepper" pattern ● Enhances with contrast.

▶ **DSA findings**
Marked contrast filling of the tumor from large arterial feeders ● Early venous filling.

Clinical Aspects

▶ **Typical presentation**
Pulsatile tinnitus ● Hearing loss because of impaired sound transmission ● Facial nerve palsy.

▶ **Therapeutic options**
Treatment of choice is microsurgical resection ● Preoperative embolization reduces intraoperative complications ● Radiation therapy.

▶ **Course and prognosis**
Radical removal is usually feasible.

▶ **What does the clinician want to know?**
Diagnosis ● Size ● Is an interventional procedure indicated?

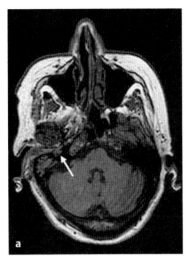

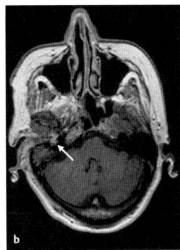

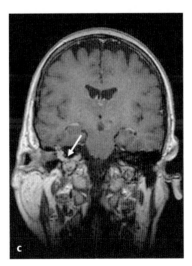

Fig. 3.5 a–c Glomus tympanicum tumor. T1-weighted MRI before (**a**) and after administration of gadolinium contrast agent (**b,c**). The tumor (arrow) in the right middle ear is isointense to brain tissue on the precontrast T1-weighted image (**a**) and shows pronounced enhancement with contrast (**b,c**).

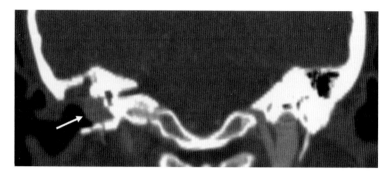

Fig. 3.6 Recurrent glomus tympanicum tumor. Unenhanced CT with coronal reconstruction. Mass (arrow) isodense to soft tissue in the right middle ear (courtesy of Dr. R. Klingebiel, Berlin).

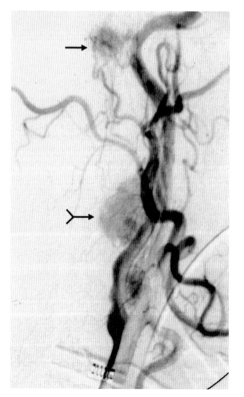

Fig. 3.7 Simultaneous occurrence of a glomus tympanicum tumor (arrow) and a carotid body tumor (serrated arrow) on DSA.

Differential Diagnosis

Aberrant internal carotid artery	– CT, CTA, and MRI show the characteristic abnormal course of the artery in the middle ear
Cholesteatoma	– Severe bony destruction – No "salt and pepper" pattern, ring enhancement only or none at all
Squamous cell carcinoma of the middle ear	– Severe bony destruction in the temporal bone, originating from the middle ear cavity and external acoustic meatus
Schwannoma of the facial nerve	– Soft tissue mass along the course of the nerve that enhances with contrast

Tips and Pitfalls

A glomus jugulare tumor can be mistaken for a glomus tympanicum tumor • An aberrant internal carotid artery can be misinterpreted as a tumor.

Selected References

van den Berg R. Imaging and management of head and neck paragangliomas. Eur Radiol 2005; 15: 1310–1318

Jackson CG. Glomus tympanicum and glomus jugulare tumors. Otolaryngol Clin North Am 2001; 34: 941–970

Rao AB et al. Paragangliomas of the head and neck: radiologic-pathologic correlation. RadioGraphics 1999; 19: 1605–1632

Glomus Jugulare Tumor

Definition

▶ **Epidemiology**
Second most common glomus tumor • Peak age of occurrence is 40–60 years • Females are affected four to six times more often than males.

▶ **Etiology, pathophysiology, pathogenesis**
Occurs in the jugular foramen and adjacent skull base • Arises from the paraganglia on the floor of the middle ear cavity immediately adjacent to the superior bulb of the jugular vein and the tympanic canaliculus • Locally destructive growth is typical • Extensive tissue defects.

Imaging Signs

▶ **Modality of choice**
CT • MRI.

▶ **CT findings**
Widening and erosion of the jugular fossa by a markedly enhancing soft tissue tumor (best evaluated in both soft tissue and bone windows) • *Directions of growth:* Laterally into the hypotympanum and middle ear with destruction of the ossicles of the middle ear, inferiorly along the internal jugular vein and caudal cranial nerves, posteriorly into the sigmoid sinus, superiorly into the inner ear and internal auditory canal, and medially into the cerebellopontine angle.

▶ **MRI findings**
Hypointense or isointense to muscle on T1-weighted images • Hyperintense on T2-weighted images • Typical but not pathognomonic findings on noncontrast sequences (especially T2-weighted) include the "salt and pepper" pattern • Marked enhancement.

▶ **DSA findings**
Tumor blush • Dilated arterial feeders • Early venous drainage • Arterial and venous collaterals • Infiltration of adjacent blood vessels.

Clinical Aspects

▶ **Typical presentation**
Pulsatile tinnitus • Hearing impairment • Impaired balance • Distal cranial nerve deficits (paresis of the soft palate, hoarseness, dysphagia, paralysis of the tongue) in late stage.

▶ **Therapeutic options**
Method of choice is surgical resection • Preoperative embolization decreases the risk of complications involving hemorrhage • Radiation therapy may be used in selected cases.

▶ **Course and prognosis**
Rate of recurrence is as high as 50% • Mortality is about 15% • Frequency of malignancy is about 3%.

▶ **What does the clinician want to know?**
Diagnosis • Size • Is embolization indicated?

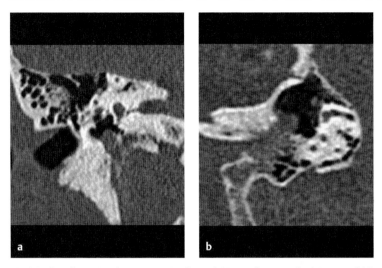

Fig. 3.8 a, b Glomus jugulare tumor. Unenhanced CT scan (bone window) in coronal (**a**) and sagittal (**b**) reconstruction. Destruction of the petrous bone structures from a soft tissue tumor that has invaded the middle ear cavity (courtesy of Dr. R. Klingebiel, Berlin).

Differential Diagnosis

Schwannoma of the jugular fossa	– Smooth widening of the jugular foramen – No "salt and pepper" pattern
Meningioma of the jugular fossa	– Sclerosis, remodeling, or, rarely, erosion of the adjacent bone – Calcifications within the tumor
Metastases of renal or thyroid carcinomas	– Bone destruction – "Salt and pepper" pattern

Tips and Pitfalls

These lesions can resemble metastases from renal and thyroid carcinoma, where findings include bone destruction and a "salt and pepper" pattern.

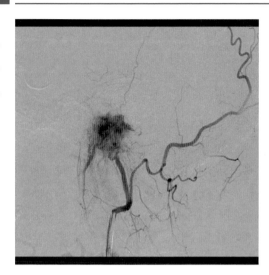

Fig. 3.9 Glomus jugulare tumor with pronounced tumor blush. DSA.

Selected References

van den Berg R. Imaging and management of head and neck paragangliomas. Eur Radiol 2005; 15: 1310–1318

Jackson CG. Glomus tympanicum and glomus jugulare tumors. Otolaryngol Clin North Am 2001; 34: 941–970

Rao AB et al. Paragangliomas of the head and neck: radiologic-pathologic correlation. RadioGraphics 1999; 19: 1605–1632

Definition

▶ **Epidemiology**
Most common glomus tumor in the head and neck region (accounting for 40% of such lesions) • Peak age is between 45 and 50 years • Equally common in males and females.

▶ **Etiology, pathophysiology, pathogenesis**
Arises from the carotid body on the posteromedial aspect of the carotid bifurcation • Incidence is increased in chronic obstructive pulmonary disorders and in inhabitants of mountain areas • Hereditary forms (about 10% of all cases) are caused by a defect in the genes that encode components of the mitochondrial oxidative pathway • Multicentric tumors occur in 15% of all cases (and in 30% of familial cases) • Associated with paragangliomas in other regions.

Imaging Signs

▶ **Modality of choice**
CT • MRI.

▶ **Color Doppler ultrasound findings**
Hypoechoic, hypervascularized mass in the carotid triangle • Carotid bifurcation is widened.

▶ **CT findings**
Sharply demarcated mass • Isodense to soft tissue • Marked enhancement.

▶ **MRI findings**
Hypointense or isointense to muscle on T1-weighted images • Hyperintense on T2-weighted images • Typical but not pathognomonic findings on noncontrast sequences (especially T2-weighted) include the "salt and pepper" pattern • Marked enhancement.

▶ **DSA findings**
Pronounced tumor enhancement • Dilated arterial feeders • Early venous drainage • May show infiltration of the internal carotid artery • Arterial and venous collaterals • Study can exclude a second tumor.

Clinical Aspects

▶ **Typical presentation**
Slow-growing painless neck tumor • Largely asymptomatic • Occasionally accompanied by dysphagia • Compression of the vagus nerve can produce hoarseness.

▶ **Therapeutic options**
Primary surgical resection • Preoperative embolization decreases the risk of complications involving hemorrhage • Palliative radiation therapy may be indicated for very extensive or recurrent tumors and to treat metastases.

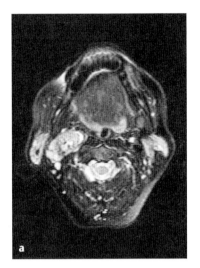

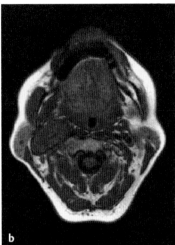

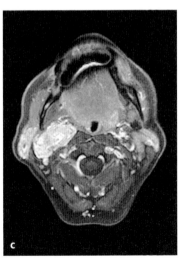

Fig. 3.10 a–c Carotid body tumor. Axial MRI. The well demarcated oval mass in the right carotid triangle is hyperintense on the T2-weighted image (**a**) and iso-intense to muscle on the noncontrasted T1-weighted image (**b**). Pronounced homogeneous enhancement after contrast administration (**c**). Particularly on the T2-weighted image (**a**), findings include areas of higher and lower signal intensity within the tumor ("salt and pepper" pattern).

▶ **Course and prognosis**
   Rate of recurrence is about 10% • Mortality is about 9% • Malignant growth occurs in 2–13% of all cases.
▶ **What does the clinician want to know?**
   Diagnosis • Size • Is an interventional procedure indicated?

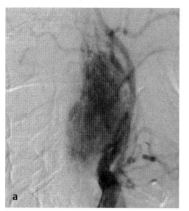
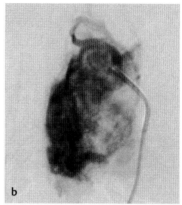

Fig. 3.11 a, b Carotid body tumor. DSA. The initial angiogram (**a**) and selective image of the ascending pharyngeal artery (**b**) demonstrate a pronounced tumor blush.

Differential Diagnosis

Abscess	– Fluid retention with ring enhancement
Lymphadenopathy	– Increased intranodal vascularity on color-coded duplex sonography
Metastases of renal or thyroid carcinomas	– Hypervascularized soft tissue masses with "salt and pepper" pattern
Schwannoma of the vagus nerve	– Anteromedial displacement of the carotid arteries and posterior displacement of the jugular vein
	– Nonspecific signal behavior on MRI

Tips and Pitfalls

Where color Doppler ultrasound detects increased intratumor vascularization, the lesion can be confused with inflammatory or malignant adenopathy • Can be misinterpreted as metastases of renal or thyroid carcinomas • Can be misinterpreted as other neoplasms of the neck, such as melanoma, angiosarcoma, or hemangiopericytoma.

Selected References

van den Berg R. Imaging and management of head and neck paragangliomas. Eur Radiol 2005; 15: 1310–1318

van der Mey AGL et al. Management of carotid body tumors. Otolaryngol Clin North Am 2001; 34: 907–924

Rao AB et al. Paragangliomas of the head and neck: radiologic-pathologic correlation. RadioGraphics 1999; 19: 1605–1632

Definition

▶ **Epidemiology**
Most common type of primary vasculitis ● Generally manifests itself after 50 years ● Peak age is between 75 and 85 years ● Prevalence in Europe and North America is 19–32 : 100 000 among people over 50 years and 49 : 100 000 among people over 80 years ● Females are affected twice as often as males.

▶ **Etiology, pathophysiology, pathogenesis**
Immunologically mediated arteritis of large- and medium-sized arteries ● Histologic picture of lymphocytic and histiocytic infiltration ● Formation of giant cell granulomas ● Intimal proliferation and fibrosis ● This leads to obstruction of the lumen in the late stage ● The disorder shows a predilection for the extracranial arteries of the head (cranial arteritis), particularly the superficial temporal artery (temporal arteritis) ● Other commonly affected arteries include the arteries of the proximal arm and leg and the aorta.

Imaging Signs

▶ **Modality of choice**
Modality of choice for demonstrating temporal arteritis is color Doppler ultrasound ● Gold standard for confirming the diagnosis is temporal arterial biopsy ● MRI is an alternative modality.

▶ **Color Doppler ultrasound findings**
Concentric, markedly hypoechoic thickening of the wall (halo) of the temporal artery (inflammatory edema of the arterial wall) ● Stenosis (peak systolic velocity increased to more than twice normal) ● Occlusion.

▶ **MRI findings**
Thickening of the arterial wall and surrounding tissue ● Strong mural enhancement on postcontrast fat-saturated T1-weighted images.

▶ **CTA, MRA and DSA findings**
Stenosis or occlusion of the proximal arteries of the extremities (subclavian, axillary, and femoral arteries) ● Aortic aneurysm and/or dissection (predilection for the thoracic aorta).

▶ **FDG-PET**
Screening modality for detecting vasculitis of the extracranial arteries.

Clinical Aspects

▶ **Typical presentation**
General symptoms: Fatigue ● Fever ● Depressive mood ● Loss of appetite ● Weight loss. *Vascular symptoms:* Temporal headache ● Tenderness to palpation and hardening over the superficial temporal artery ● Claudication of the jaws ● Impaired vision including blindness ● Claudication in the extremities ● Cerebral insult ● Myocardial infarction ● *Symptoms of polymyalgia rheumatica* (in about 50% of all cases): Muscle pain in the neck, shoulder girdle, and pelvis ● Labora-

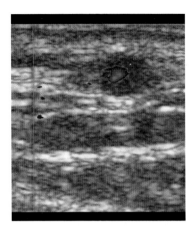

Fig. 3.12 Giant cell arteritis. Color Doppler ultrasound. Hypoechoic thickening of the wall (halo) of the superficial temporal artery seen in cross section. The thickness of the halo (distance marks) is 0.7 mm.

tory findings include elevated erythrocyte sedimentation rate (> 50 mm/h) and C-reactive protein levels.

▸ **Therapeutic options**

Glucocorticoids • Radiologic intervention • Surgical management.

▸ **Course and prognosis**

Responds well to steroids.

▸ **What does the clinician want to know?**

Extent and activity of the vascular process • Exclude extracranial carotid stenosis prior to temporal arterial biopsy as the superficial temporal artery can be part of an extracranial–intracranial collateral system.

Differential Diagnosis

Takayasu arteritis	– Age under 40
	– Usually affects the aortic arch and its primary branches
Atherosclerosis	– Wall thickening is more hyperechoic and irregular

Tips and Pitfalls

Very peripheral involvement of the temporal artery can produce false-negative findings on color Doppler ultrasound, being beyond the limit of spatial resolution • False-negative findings are also possible in the absence of a halo where there is only partial infiltration of the vascular wall in the early phase of the disorder, or where the halo has receded in response to steroid therapy.

Selected References

Bley TA et al. [MRI in giant cell (temporal) arteritis.] Rofo 2007; 179: 703–711 [In German]
Bley TA et al. High-resolution MRI in giant-cell arteritis: imaging of the wall of the superficial temporal artery. AJR Am J Roentgenol 2005; 184: 283–287

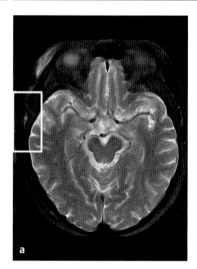

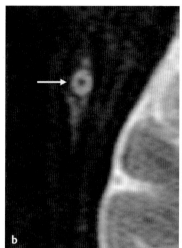

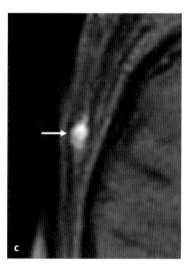

Fig. 3.13 a–c Giant cell arteritis. Axial MRI. **a, b** Fat-suppressed T2-weighted sequence. The entire circumference of the neurocranium is visualized at the level of the temporal lobe (**a**), as is a section of the right extracranial temporal region (**b**). Concentric thickening of the wall of the right superficial temporal artery (arrow) and surrounding edema. **c** Same view on a fat-suppressed T1-weighted image after administration of gadolinium contrast. Pronounced homogeneous enhancement is seen in the thickened arterial wall.

Schmidt WA, Blockmans D. Use of ultrasonography and positron emission tomography in the diagnosis and assessment of large-vessel vasculitis. Curr Opin Rheumatol 2005; 17: 9–15

Weyand CM, Goronzy JJ. Giant-cell arteritis and polymyalgia rheumatica. Ann Intern Med 2003; 139: 505–515

Definition

▶ **Epidemiology**
Accounts for less than 5% of all cases of deep venous thrombosis.

▶ **Etiology, pathophysiology, pathogenesis**
Central venous catheter • Implantation of cardiac pacemaker • Surgery • Bacterial oropharyngeal infection • Cellulitis or abscess in the neck • Intravenous drug use • Paraneoplastic symptom • Coagulatory disorders (protein C and S deficiency, polycythemia vera) • Hormonal causes (pregnancy, hormone therapy) • Traumatic causes (rare).

Imaging Signs

▶ **Modality of choice**
Color Doppler ultrasound.

▶ **Color Doppler ultrasound findings**
Dilated noncompressible lumen with hypoechoic internal echo pattern • Lumen does not fluctuate with respiration • Absence of flow signs • Venous collateralization.

▶ **CT findings**
Unenhanced scan shows a dilated hyperdense lumen • Minimally enhancing thrombus is visualized after contrast administration • There may be a hyperdense halo of blood around the thrombus • Venous wall may be hypervascularized • Surrounding tissue may show reactive changes.

▶ **MRI findings**
Flow signal is absent on MR venography • Thrombus incompletely blocking blood flow may be demonstrated.

Clinical Aspects

▶ **Typical presentation**
Often asymptomatic or showing only nonspecific symptoms • Neck swelling • Headache • Enlarged cervical lymph nodes • Fever • In inflammatory cases, symptoms may progress to the clinical picture of sepsis.

▶ **Therapeutic options**
Initial therapy includes intravenous antibiotics and systemic heparinization • This is followed by anticoagulation over 3–6 months • Surgery is indicated where complications occur.

▶ **Course and prognosis**
Prognosis depends on the underlying disorder • Numerous complications may occur • Abscess • Sepsis with septic embolization • Ascending thrombosis as far as the intracranial vessels • Pulmonary embolism • Endocarditis • Meningitis • Disseminated intravascular coagulation.

▶ **What does the clinician want to know?**
Extent • Complications.

Fig. 3.14   Acute thrombosis of the internal jugular vein. Color Doppler ultrasound. The lumen of the vein is completely occluded by hypoechoic thrombotic material.

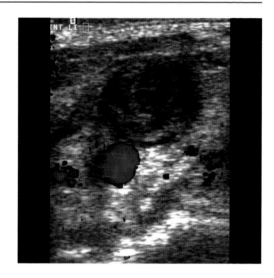

Differential Diagnosis

Abscess	– Fluid retention with ring enhancement and occasionally central gas inclusions (contrast-enhanced CT)
Inflammatory or malignant adenopathy	– Usually multiple round hypoechoic masses showing marked enhancement (CT, MRI), occasionally with intranodal vascularization (color Doppler ultrasound)

Tips and Pitfalls

Can be confused with an abscess.

Selected References

Boedeker CC et al. [Etiology and therapy of the internal jugular vein thrombosis.] Laryngorhinootologie 2004; 83: 743–749 [In German]

Sheikh MA et al. Isolated internal jugular vein thrombosis: risk factors and natural history. Vasc Med 2002; 7: 177–179

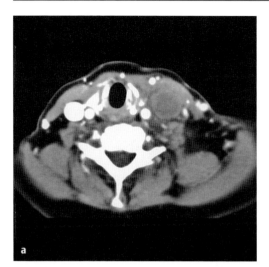

Fig. 3.15 a, b Contrast-enhanced CT shows acute thrombotic occlusion of the left internal jugular vein. **a** Transverse image. **b** Coronal reconstruction.

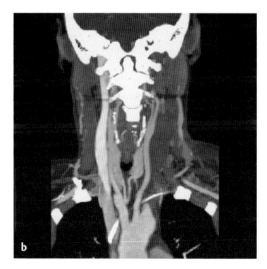

Definition

▶ **Epidemiology**
Prevalence of carotid artery stenosis exceeding 50% is 7% in people over 65 years • The risk of ischemic cerebral infarction attributable to carotid artery stenosis is 1–2% per year where stenosis is greater than 50% and 2–5% per year where stenosis is greater than 80% • Extracranial carotid stenosis or occlusion is responsible for about 20% of all ischemic insults in the anterior cerebrovascular system • There is a significant association with coronary artery disease and peripheral occlusive arterial disease.

▶ **Etiology, pathophysiology, pathogenesis**
The most common cause (> 90% of all cases) is atherosclerosis • Less common causes include fibromuscular dysplasia, dissection, radiation-induced carotid lesions, recurrent stenoses secondary to endarterectomy • *Risk factors:* Age, sex, positive family history, hypertension, smoking, diabetes mellitus, and hyperlipidemia • Atherosclerotic carotid stenoses show a predilection for the carotid bulb and the origin of the internal carotid artery • Tandem stenoses are present in 2% of all cases • The underlying cause of cerebral ischemia due to compromise of the carotid artery is usually an arterial embolism of plaque and thrombus material • Hemodynamic infarcts are rare (< 10% of all cases).

Imaging Signs

▶ **Modality of choice**
Color Doppler ultrasound • MRA • CTA.

▶ **Color Doppler ultrasound findings**
Partially calcified plaques (acoustic shadows) or ulcerated marginal plaques may be present • Narrowed lumen • Proportional flow acceleration • Poststenotic turbulence and dilation.

▶ **CT findings**
Findings include sequelae of ischemia (leukoencephalopathy, infarcts).

▶ **CTA findings**
Calcifications are better visualized than on MRI.

▶ **MRI findings**
Findings include sequelae of ischemia.

▶ **MRA findings**
Demonstrates stenosis • Severity of the stenosis can be overestimated.

▶ **DSA**
This allows the most accurate estimation of the severity of the stenosis • Intervention is then possible (stent placement or balloon dilation and protection) • Postinterventional follow-up.

Table 3.1 Parameters for quantifying carotid artery stenosis on color Doppler ultrasound (adapted from Grant et al.)

Degree of stenosis	Parameters
< 50%	ICA-MSV < 125 cm/s MSV ratio ICA/CCA < 2 ICA-EDV < 40 cm/s
50–69%	ICA-MSV 125–230 cm/s MSV ratio ICA/CCA 2–4 ICA-EDV 40–100 cm/s
≥ 70% but less than near occlusion	ICA-MSV > 230 cm/s MSV ratio ICA/CCA > 4 ICA-EDV > 100 cm/s
Near occlusion	ICA-MSV high, low, or not detectable Additional parameters (MSV ratio, ICA-EDV) are variable
Complete occlusion	ICA-MSV not detectable Additional parameters not applicable

ICA = internal carotid artery; CCA = common carotid artery; EDV = end-diastolic velocity; MSV = maximum systolic velocity.

Clinical Aspects

▶ **Typical presentation**
  Asymptomatic ● Transient ischemic attacks ● Cerebral ischemic infarction.
▶ **Therapeutic options**
  Therapy is indicated only for symptomatic stenosis where the lumen is narrowed over 70% ● Current studies show that endarterectomy leads to slightly better outcome than stent placement.
▶ **Course and prognosis**
  This depends on patient compliance and on treatment of the underlying disease ● Progressive.
▶ **What does the clinician want to know?**
  Extent of the stenosis ● Other causes of the symptoms.

Differential Diagnosis

Extraluminal compression of the carotid artery	– Clearly detectable on CT and MRI
Dissection	– No calcifications

Fig. 3.16 a, b Extracranial carotid artery stenosis. Color Doppler ultrasound. High-grade stenosis of the internal carotid artery with local flow acceleration, detectable as aliasing. Abnormal Doppler spectrum at the stenosis with increased systolic and diastolic velocity.

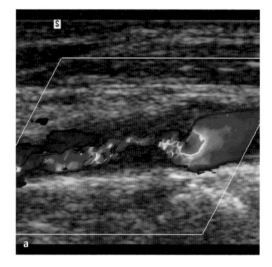

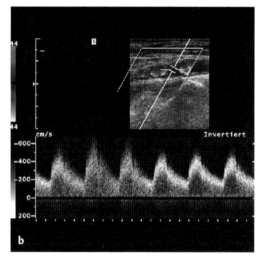

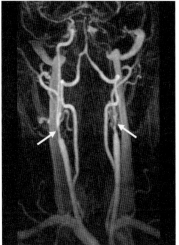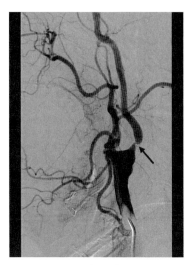

Fig. 3.17 Bolus contrast-enhanced MRA. Bilateral stenoses at the origin of each internal carotid artery (arrows).

Fig. 3.18 DSA. High-grade stenosis (arrow) of the left internal carotid artery.

Tips and Pitfalls

Incorrect examination technique with color Doppler ultrasound, such as Doppler angle > 60°, inadequate pulse repetition frequency, incorrect placement of the Doppler range gate ● Complicating anatomic factors include a high carotid bifurcation (short neck), vascular tortuosity or formation of vascular slings, shadows created by calcification plaques, and tandem stenoses ● The severity of the stenosis is easy to overestimate on MRI.

Selected References

Eckstein HH et al. Surgical therapy of extracranial carotid stenosis. Chirurg 2004; 75: 93–110 [In German]

Grant EG et al. Carotid artery stenosis: gray-scale and Doppler US diagnosis—Society of Radiologists in Ultrasound consensus conference. Radiology 2003; 229: 340–346

Lell M et al. Evaluation of carotid artery stenosis with multisection CT and MR imaging: influence of imaging modality and postprocessing. AJNR Am J Neuroradiol 2007; 28: 104–110

Mas JL, EVA-3S Investigators. Endarterectomy versus stenting in patients with symptomatic severe carotid stenosis. N Engl J Med 2006; 355: 1660–1671

Nederkoorn PJ et al. Overestimation of carotid artery stenosis with magnetic resonance angiography compared with digital subtraction angiography. J Vasc Surg 2002; 36: 806–813

Definition

▶ **Epidemiology**
Incidence rate in the USA is 2–3 : 100 000 per year • Second most common cause of cerebral infarction in patients under 45 years (accounting for 10–25 % in this age group) • It is the cause of insult in about 2 % of all cases in all age groups • Females are affected 1.5 times as often as males • Peak age for spontaneous dissections is 40–45.

▶ **Etiology, pathophysiology, pathogenesis**
Confirmed risk factors include hereditary connective tissue disorders such as Ehlers–Danlos syndrome type IV and Marfan syndrome • Uncertain risk factors include fibromuscular dysplasia, migraine, homocystinuria, oral contraceptive use, chronic infection, and arterial hypertension • Traumatic dissection may occur after cranial trauma, cervical vertebral fracture, strangulation, or hanging • Iatrogenic causes include chiropractic maneuvers, angiography, angioplasty, and overextension of the neck in intubation.

– Tear of the vascular intima or rupture of the vasa vasorum • Both cases give rise to a hematoma expanding within the tunica media • The often eccentric location of the hematoma either leads to obstruction of the lumen (subintimal dissection) or formation of a pseudoaneurysm (subadventitial dissection) • Dissection most often occurs in the segment of the artery from 2 cm to 3 cm distal to the bifurcation to the skull base • It rarely occurs in the petrous or cavernous segment of the carotid artery.

Imaging Signs

▶ **Modality of choice**
MRI • MRA • CTA.

▶ **Color Doppler ultrasound findings**
Occasionally there will be direct signs of dissection: tapering stenosis, intramural hematoma (hypoechoic mass in the vascular wall), double lumen, intimal flap • Indirect signs include abnormal Doppler spectra (peripheral increase in resistance up to and including complete interruption of blood flow) • Monitoring the course of hemodynamics after dissection.

▶ **CTA findings**
Stenosis or occlusion of the artery • Intramural hematoma • Artery is dilated with a narrower perivascular fat layer than in the contralateral artery.

▶ **MRI findings**
Absent or eccentrically reduced flow void • Crescent-shape widened vascular wall with a hyperintense signal on axial T2-weighted and T1-weighted sequences after fat suppression from about the third day to a maximum of 6–9 months after the dissection • The initial intramural hematoma is often hypointense on T2-weighted and T1-weighted images • Diffusion and perfusion imaging demonstrate cerebral ischemia.

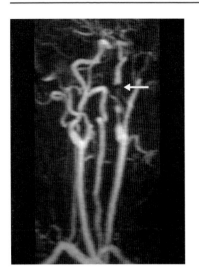

Fig. 3.19 Subintimal carotid artery dissection. MIP reconstruction of a contrast-enhanced MRA. Focal dilation followed by high-grade stenosis of the left internal carotid artery (arrow).

▸ **MRA findings**
Irregularities of the lumen including complete occlusion ● Development of a pseudoaneurysm.

▸ **DSA findings**
Now only rarely indicated in acute cases ● "String sign" (long stretch of narrowed lumen) ● Tapered proximal occlusion (flame-shaped occlusion) ● Pseudoaneurysm.

Clinical Aspects

▸ **Typical presentation**
Neck pain (anterolateral, radiating into the angle of the mandible or behind the ear) ● Headache (frontal and retroorbital) ● Pulsatile tinnitus ● Symptoms of transient ischemic attack (amaurosis fugax, aphasia) ● Peripheral Horner syndrome ● Cranial nerve deficits (cranial nerves III–XII), most commonly involving the lowest cranial nerves, especially the hypoglossal nerve ● Cerebral infarct (primarily embolic, less often hemodynamic) ● Asymptomatic in only 5% of all cases.

▸ **Therapeutic options**
Anticoagulation ● Rarely surgery or stenting.

▸ **Course and prognosis**
With anticoagulation treatment the lesion usually resolves completely or nearly completely within the first few months ● Mortality is 5%, morbidity 25%.

▸ **What does the clinician want to know?**
Confirm the dissection ● Prognostic estimation ● Follow-up during and after therapy.

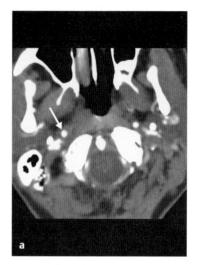 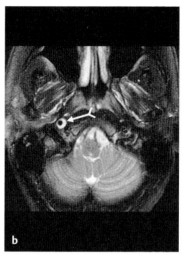

Fig. 3.20 a, b Subadventitial carotid artery dissection.
a Axial CTA. Circumferential thickening, isodense to soft tissue, of the wall (arrow) of the right internal carotid artery. The vascular lumen is intact.
b Axial T-weighted MRI with fat suppression (axial slices). Crescentic hyperintense intramural hematoma (forked arrow). The lumen exhibits a normal flow void.

Differential Diagnosis

Atherosclerosis	– Involves the carotid bifurcation and the carotid bulb
	– Typical calcification pattern
Thrombosis	– Thrombus can usually be identified after contrast administration
Fibromuscular dysplasia	– Irregular narrowing of a long stretch of the internal carotid resembling a string of pearls

Tips and Pitfalls

In a subadventitial hematoma without any reduction in the lumen, the dissection can be overlooked on CTA • Hematoma in the vascular wall is often hard to identify on MRI within the first 24–48 hours after the dissection because of its low signal intensity; failure to use fat suppression on T1-weighted sequences is a common error.

Selected References

Brandt T et al. Clinical treatment and therapy for dissected cervicocerebral artery. Nerven-arzt 2006; 77: S17–30 [In German]

Chandra A et al. Spontaneous dissection of the carotid and vertebral arteries: the 10-year UCSD Experience. Ann Vasc Surg 2007; 21: 178–185

Flis CM et al. Carotid and vertebral artery dissections: clinical aspects, imaging features and endovascular treatment. Eur Radiol 2007; 17: 820–834

Schievink WI. Current concepts: spontaneous dissection of the carotid and vertebral arteries. N Engl J Med 2001; 344: 898–906

Definition

▶ **Epidemiology**
Estimated incidence rate is 1–1.5 : 100 000 per year.

▶ **Etiology, pathophysiology, pathogenesis**
Known risk factors include hereditary connective tissue disorders such as Marfan syndrome and Ehlers–Danlos syndrome type IV • Uncertain risk factors include fibromuscular dysplasia, migraine, homocystinuria, oral contraceptive use, chronic infection, and arterial hypertension • Traumatic dissection may occur after cranial trauma, cervical vertebral fracture, direct vascular injury, strangulation, or hanging • Iatrogenic causes include chiropractic maneuvers, angiography, angioplasty, and overextension of the neck in intubation.

Tear of the vascular intima or rupture of the vasa vasorum • Both cases give rise to a hematoma expanding within the tunica media • The often eccentric location of the hematoma leads either to obstruction of the lumen (subintimal dissection) or formation of a pseudoaneurysm (subadventitial dissection) • Dissection most often occurs in the distal arterial loop at the atlas (V3 segment) • It occurs less often in the prevertebral segment of the artery (V1 segment).

Imaging Signs

▶ **Modality of choice**
MRI • MRA • CTA.

▶ **Color Doppler ultrasound findings**
The direct and indirect Doppler criteria for detecting dissection are less sensitive in the vertebral artery than in the internal carotid artery.

▶ **CT findings**
Demonstrates subarachnoid hemorrhage where the dissection extends into the cranium.

▶ **CTA findings**
Stenosis or occlusion of the artery • Intramural hematoma • Artery is dilated with a narrower perivascular fat layer than in the contralateral artery.

▶ **MRI findings**
Fat-suppressed T1-weighted and T2-weighted images show a hyperintense halo • The flow void is normal or reduced.

▶ **MRA findings**
Given the smaller diameter and the physiologic fluctuations in caliber, MRA findings are more difficult to interpret than in the internal carotid artery.

▶ **DSA findings**
Irregular narrowing of the lumen that begins gradually • Pseudoaneurysm (25 % of all cases) • Intimal flap and double lumen (10 % of all cases).

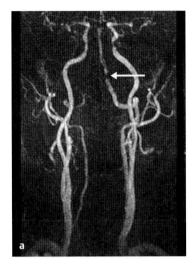

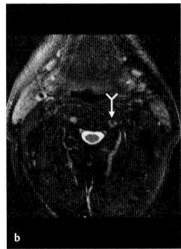

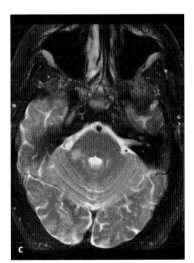

Fig. 3.21 a–c Vertebral artery dissection. **a** Postcontrast MRA. Short high-grade stenosis of the left vertebral artery in segment V4 (arrow). Hypoplastic right vertebral artery. **b** T2-weighted axial MRI. Hyperintense collar (forked arrow) in the wall of the left vertebral artery. **c** MRI, T2-weighted image. Infarct in the right brainstem measuring about 1 cm.

Clinical Aspects

▶ **Typical presentation**
Neck pain (posterolateral) • Headache (back of the head and neck) • Symptoms of transient ischemic attack (vertigo, nausea, optic ataxia, unsteady gait) • Central Horner syndrome • Brainstem ischemia (in about 50% of all cases) • Dissection in segment V4 may result in subarachnoid hemorrhage.

▶ **Therapeutic options**
Anticoagulation • Where clinical symptoms persist or embolic events occur, surgical ligation or endovascular occlusion may be indicated.

▶ **Course and prognosis**
Spontaneous healing • In 90% of all cases the stenosis significantly decreases or resolves entirely within 3 months • Rate of recurrence is 8%, usually within the first month • Subarachnoid hemorrhage is rare.

▶ **What does the clinician want to know?**
Confirm the dissection • Prognostic estimation • Follow-up during and after therapy.

Differential Diagnosis

Atherosclerosis	– Findings often include calcified plaques
Fibromuscular dysplasia	– Imaging findings resemble a string of pearls; very rare

Tips and Pitfalls

A pseudohematoma produced by slow blood flow in the periarterial venous plexus can mimic a vertebral artery dissection.

Selected References

Provenzale JM et al. Spontaneous vertebral dissection: clinical, conventional angiographic, CT, and MR findings. J Comput Assist Tomogr 1996; 20: 185–193

Saeed A al. Vertebral artery dissection: warning symptoms, clinical features and prognosis in 26 patients. Can J Neurol Sci 2000; 27: 292–296

Yamada M et al. Intracranial vertebral artery dissection with subarachnoid hemorrhage: clinical characteristics and outcomes in conservatively treated patients. J Neurosurg 2004; 101: 25–30

Definition

▶ **Epidemiology**

A steal syndrome is demonstrated in 1.5–6% of all cervical vascular examinations • Additional cervical arterial stenosis is present in 80% of all cases • Neurologic symptoms are present in only 5% of all cases. • Predilection for the left side (85% of all cases).

▶ **Etiology, pathophysiology, pathogenesis**

This is a special case of impaired cerebrovascular perfusion • The underlying cause is usually atherosclerosis • Pathologic changes in the arterial wall lead to plaque formation • This leads to increasing stenosis and occlusion of the left subclavian artery (85% of all cases) or the brachiocephalic trunk (15% of all cases) proximal to the origin of the vertebral artery • Persistent or intermittent retrograde flow occurs in the ipsilateral vertebral artery • Blood is drawn from the posterior cerebral flow tract, especially during intensive use of the arm • The result is cerebral ischemia.

Imaging Signs

▶ **Modality of choice**

Color Doppler ultrasound.

▶ **General findings**

Narrowing of the lumen of the subclavian artery compared with the proximal or distal segment, or occlusion • Calcifications are often present • Retrograde flow in the vertebral artery.

▶ **Color Doppler ultrasound findings**

Retrograde flow in the vertebral artery in combination with a poststenotic spectrum in the brachial artery • In low-grade stenosis at rest there will be diminished or oscillating flow (biphasic Doppler signals) in the vertebral artery • Provocation (arm exercise or pressure cuff) will then produce retrograde flow • The carotid bifurcation can also be visualized • Supplementary diagnostic studies are indicated prior to interventional or surgical treatment.

▶ **CTA**

Technical requirements include multidetector CT and rapid injection of contrast agent • The aortic arch and intracerebral arteries are evaluated • The stenosis is directly visualized after contrast injection • A dynamic examination with visualization of retrograde flow is possible by measuring a test bolus in the neck • Vascular calcification can be readily evaluated.

▶ **MRA**

Technical requirements include a head coil and contrast-enhanced MRA with rapid data acquisition • The aortic arch, cervical arteries, and intracerebral arteries are evaluated • Retrograde flow is visualized by serial measurements, for example with parallel imaging and a keyhole technique • Alternatives include phase-contrast and time-of-flight techniques.

Fig. 3.22   Subclavian steal syndrome.

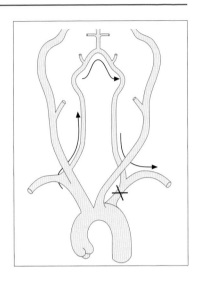

► **DSA**

This is indicated only where CTA or MRA of sufficient quality is unavailable and where percutaneous treatment is planned.

Clinical Aspects

► **Typical presentation**

Weakened or absent pulse in the left hand • Blood pressure difference between the right and left arms (> 20 mmHg) • Often asymptomatic • Symptoms occur only in the presence of additional stenosis and/or occlusion • These then include vertigo, nausea, and impaired vision • Use of the arm rarely exacerbates symptoms, but this finding is typical where it does occur • Ischemia of the hand with pain during exercise or at rest is rare.

► **Therapeutic options**

Angioplasty, possibly with stent placement, is indicated only in symptomatic cases • Alternatives include vascular surgery (usually a bypass procedure).

► **Course and prognosis**

Subclavian steal is usually asymptomatic • 5-year patency rate after revascularization is over 85%.

► **What does the clinician want to know?**

Visualization and evaluation of all cervical vessels and the intracerebral vessels as well.

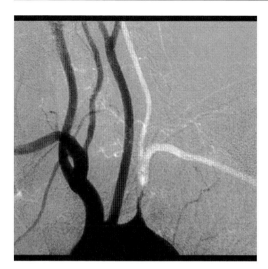

Fig. 3.23 High-grade stenosis of the subclavian artery with retrograde flow in the vertebral artery. DSA of the aortic arch and supra-aortic arteries. Setting the DSA mask after the initial passage of contrast agent (black) visualizes the vertebral artery (perfused later and retrogradely) and subclavian arteries in white.

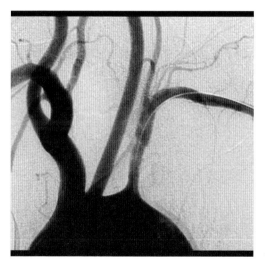

Fig. 3.24 DSA after percutaneous balloon angioplasty treatment nows shows physiologic flow in the vertebral artery.

Differential Diagnosis

Acute vascular occlusion (embolism, dissection)	– Sudden onset – Abrupt vascular occlusion – Slight atherosclerotic changes in the vascular wall
Vasculitis	– Usually younger patients
Thoracic stent graft	– Occlusion of the origin of the subclavian artery is occasionally necessary to completely eliminate a thoracic aneurysm (history)

Tips and Pitfalls

Failure to investigate incidental findings with CTA or MRA.

Selected References

Buckenham TM, Wright IA. Ultrasound of the extracranial vertebral artery. Br J Radiol 2004; 77: 15–20

Wu C et al. Subclavian steal syndrome: diagnosis with perfusion metrics from contrast-enhanced MR angiographic bolus-timing examination—initial experience. Radiology 2005; 235: 927–933

Chest

Definition

▶ **Epidemiology**
Occurs in 0.3–0.5% of the population • Occurs in 11% of patients with congenital heart defects.

▶ **Etiology, pathophysiology, pathogenesis**
Persistence of the left anterior cardinal vein inferior to the origin of the brachiocephalic vein • This leads to persistence of the left superior vena cava draining into the right atrium via the coronary sinus • The communicating vessel between the two superior venae cavae (left brachiocephalic vein) may be present or absent.

Imaging Signs

▶ **Modality of choice**
Incidental finding.

▶ **CT and MRI findings**
The left superior vena cava courses inferiorly to the heart at the level of the left brachiocephalic vein lateral to the aortic arch and anterior to the left main bronchus.

Clinical Aspects

▶ **Typical presentation**
Asymptomatic.

▶ **Therapeutic options**
None.

▶ **Course and prognosis**
In cases where the vein drains into the left atrium, development of a right-to-left shunt can lead to brain abscesses and peripheral thromboembolic disease.

▶ **What does the clinician want to know?**
Important in cardiac catheterization and heart surgery.

Differential Diagnosis

Anomalous drainage of the left superior pulmonary vein into the left brachiocephalic vein	– Superior pulmonary vein absent anterior to the left main bronchus – Narrow coronary sinus

Tips and Pitfalls

Be aware of possible associated malformations (such as an atrioventricular septal defect or transposition of the pulmonary veins).

Fig. 4.1 Duplication of the superior vena cava. Illustration shows a small left brachiocephalic vein connecting two superior venae cavae.

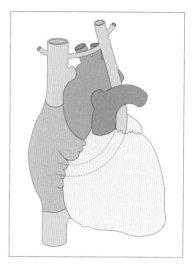

Selected References

Buirski G et al. Superior vena caval abnormalities: their occurrence rate, associated cardiac abnormalities and angiographic classification in a paediatric population with congenital heart disease. Clin Radiol 1986; 37: 131–138

Dillon EH, Camputaro C. Partial anomalous pulmonary venous drainage of the left upper lobe vs duplication of the superior vena cava: distinction based on CT findings. AJR Am J Roentgenol 1993; 160: 375–379

Minniti S et al. Congenital anomalies of the venae cavae: embryological origin, imaging features and report of three new variants. Eur Radiol 2002; 12: 2040–2055

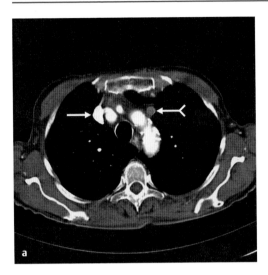

Fig. 4.2 a–c CT after contrast administration via the right arm. Axial source image (**a**) and coronal (**b**) and sagittal (**c**) reformations. The right superior vena cava (arrow) is significantly more enhanced than the left one (forked arrow).

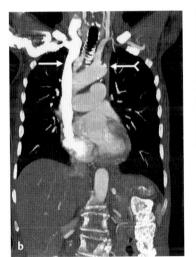

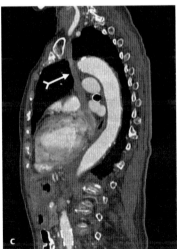

Definition

▶ **Epidemiology**
Accounts for less than 1% of all congenital defects.

▶ **Etiology, pathophysiology, pathogenesis**
Persistence of the right posterior aorta ● Two arches arise from the ascending aorta, forming a vascular ring around the trachea and esophagus ● The two arches then join together to form a single descending aorta ● Associated malformations are rare (such as tetralogy of Fallot or transposition of the great arteries) ● A genetic defect (microdeletion at 22q11) is present in some cases.

Imaging Signs

▶ **Modality of choice**
CT and MRI including contrast-enhanced MRA.

▶ **CT and MRI findings**
Both modalities provide anatomically precise visualization of the aortic arch anomaly, rendering DSA and esophagography largely obsolete ● The right arch, coursing posterior to the trachea and esophagus, is usually larger than the left one ● The left arch, coursing anterior to the trachea and esophagus, is often atretic ● The descending aorta usually lies on the left.

Clinical Aspects

▶ **Typical presentation**
The condition usually manifests itself in early infancy ● Occasionally the anomaly may remain asymptomatic until adulthood ● Abnormal breathing ● Stridor ● Frequent infections ● Apnea ● Feeding problems ● Dysphagia and dyspnea during physical exertion are the most common symptoms in adults.

▶ **Therapeutic options**
Surgical correction.

▶ **Course and prognosis**
Complete postoperative resolution of the symptoms can be achieved in most cases.

▶ **What does the clinician want to know?**
Type of aortic arch anomaly ● Identification of the dominant aortic arch ● Associated vascular variations and cardiovascular malformations.

Differential Diagnosis

Right aortic arch with retroesophageal segment	– The normal ductus arteriosus and the left descending aorta or left arteria lusoria form a vascular ring
Pulmonary artery loop	– The left pulmonary artery arises from the right pulmonary artery and courses to the left lung between the trachea and esophagus

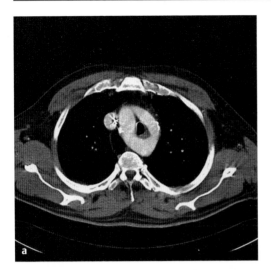

Fig. 4.3 a–c Adult patient with duplication of the aortic arch. CT after contrast administration. Axial source images (**a, b**) and volume rendering technique (**c**). The two aortic arches have formed a complete vascular ring around the esophagus and trachea (**a, c**). The four brachiocephalic arteries (**b**, arrows) usually arise separately from the ipsilateral arch segment (four-artery sign).

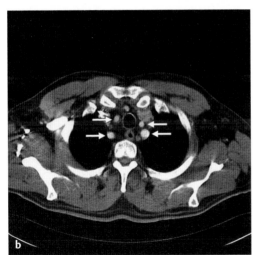

Fig. 4.3 c ▶

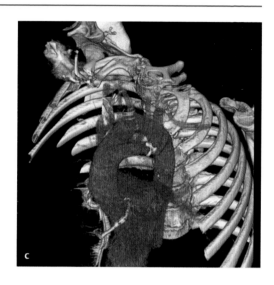

Tips and Pitfalls

In the presence of atresia of the left aortic arch, the condition is difficult to distinguish from a right aortic arch with a retroesophageal segment.

Selected References

Donnelly LF et al. The spectrum of extrinsic lower airway compression in children: MR imaging. AJR Am J Roentgenol 1997; 168: 59–62

Grathwohl MKW et al. Vascular rings of the thoracic aorta in adults. Am Surg 1999; 65: 1077–1083

Lowe GM et al. Vascular rings: 10-year review of imaging. RadioGraphics 1991; 11: 637–646

Definition

▸ **Synonym**
Arteria lusoria.

▸ **Epidemiology**
Most common anomaly of the aortic arch • Found in 0.4–2% of all autopsies.

▸ **Etiology, pathophysiology, pathogenesis**
Atresia of the fourth branchial arterial arch and the right posterior aorta up to the origin of the seventh right segmental artery • As a result, the right subclavian artery arises via the remaining distal portion of the right posterior aorta as the last branch from the aortic arch • In 80% of all cases, it courses posterior to the esophagus • In 15%, it courses between the esophagus and trachea • In 5%, it courses anterior to the trachea or main bronchi • It may arise from an aortic diverticulum (Kommerell diverticulum) • It occurs in combination with congenital heart defects (such as tetralogy of Fallot; ventricular septum defect, persistent ductus arteriosus, or coarctation of the aorta) and Down syndrome.

Imaging Signs

▸ **Modality of choice**
Usually an incidental finding.

▸ **CT and MRI findings**
Aberrant left subclavian artery arising as the last major artery from the aortic arch • It usually courses to the right, posterior to the esophagus, forming an incomplete vascular ring with the left aortic arch.

Clinical Aspects

▸ **Typical presentation**
Usually clinically occult • Dysphagia (rare).

▸ **Therapeutic options**
Surgery is indicated only in the presence of aneurysm.

▸ **Course and prognosis**
Dysphagia may also occur in late adulthood.

▸ **What does the clinician want to know?**
Esophageal compression • Association with cardiac anomalies.

Differential Diagnosis

Right aortic arch with aberrant left subclavian artery	– The aberrant left subclavian artery arises as the fourth and last artery from the right aortic arch and courses to the left, posterior to the esophagus
Duplication of the aortic arch	– The artery passing posterior to the esophagus is the right part of the vascular ring formed by the two aortic arches

Fig. 4.4 Aberrant right subclavian artery. Illustration shows the right subclavian artery arising as the last vessel from the aortic arch and coursing posterior to the trachea and esophagus.

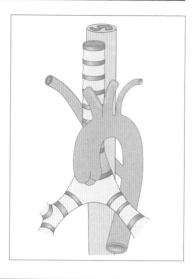

Fig. 4.5 a–c CT after contrast administration. Visualization of the right subclavian artery (arrow) on transverse source images (**a, b**) and on the oblique MIP (**c**). Shown here is a further variant in which a left vertebral artery (**b**, curved arrow) arises directly from the aortic arch and is visible between the left common carotid and left subclavian arteries.

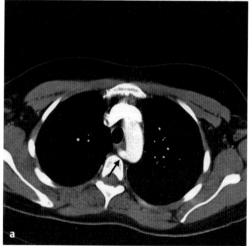

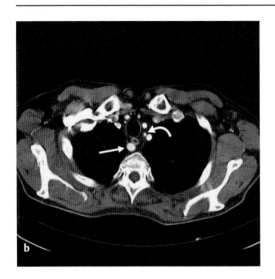

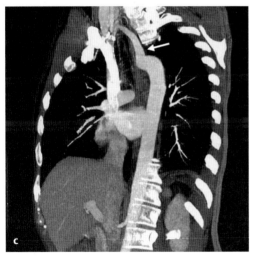

Tips and Pitfalls

Remember that this anomaly occurs relatively often in combination with coarctation of the aorta.

Selected References

Freed K, Low VHS. The aberrant subclavian artery. AJR Am J Roentgenol 1997; 168: 481–484

Donnelly LF et al. Aberrant subclavian arteries: cross-sectional imaging findings in infants and children referred for evaluation of extrinsic airway compression. AJR Am J Roentgenol 2002; 178: 1269–1274

Definition

▶ **Epidemiology**

Accounts for 7% of all congenital heart defects ● Males are affected 1.5 times as often as females ● Occurs as an isolated anomaly in 82% of all cases ● In 18% of all cases, it occurs in combination with other cardiovascular malformations (such as ventricular septum defect, hypoplastic left heart syndrome, transposition of the great arteries, hypoplasia of the aortic arch, arteria lusoria) ● Nowadays the condition is usually diagnosed prenatally ● As a result, the anomaly is generally treated at an early age and very rarely in adults.

▶ **Etiology, pathophysiology, pathogenesis**

Short congenital stenosis of the aorta at the level of the ductus arteriosus ● Location may be preductal, juxtaductal, or postductal ● Arterial hypertension in the upper half of the body results from hypoperfusion of the kidneys.

– *Adult coarctation:* Compensated by extensive collaterals (especially intercostal arteries) often into adulthood ● Usually an isolated juxtaductal or postductal form ● Late sequelae include hypertrophy of the left ventricle, cardiac failure, aortic rupture, and cerebral hemorrhage.

– *Infantile coarctation:* Severe course ● Heart failure may occur in newborns ● Coarctation is usually preductal or postductal, rarely juxtaductal ● Additional cardiac anomalies are present in 79% of all cases.

Imaging Signs

▶ **Modality of choice**

Echocardiography is used for initial diagnosis and follow-up examinations in infants ● MRI is a supplementary modality in older children and adults.

▶ **Standard chest radiograph findings**

Inverted three or epsilon sign: Infolding of the contour of the descending aorta inferior to the aortic arch ● Rib notching of the lower margin of the third to eight ribs is first seen at the age of 8–10 ● The infantile type is associated with massive cardiomegaly and signs of acute cardiac failure.

▶ **Echocardiography findings**

Stenosis is visualized ● Grade of stenosis is estimated with Doppler ● Aliasing results in a tendency to overestimate the grade of stenosis ● The aortic arch may be hypoplastic ● Associated cardiac malformations are readily identified ● Visualization of the coarctation may be limited in older children and adults ● Infantile coarctation exhibits signs of beginning cardiac insufficiency (dilation of the left ventricle, mitral valve insufficiency) and a left-to-right shunt through the distended foramen ovale.

▶ **MRI and MRA findings**

Stenosis is visualized ● Grade of stenosis can be determined ● The aortic arch may be hypoplastic ● Collaterals (intercostal arteries, internal mammary arteries, epigastric arteries, anterior spinal artery) ● Associated cardiac malformations are readily identified.

Fig. 4.6   Adult coarctation of the aorta in a 16-year-old patient. Standard chest radiograph. Typical rib notching (arrows) and abnormally configured aortic arch.

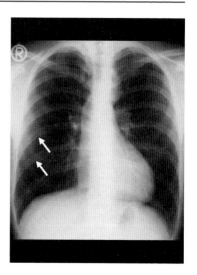

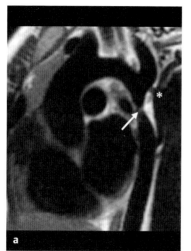

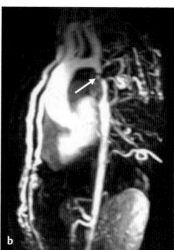

Fig. 4.7 a, b   Coarctation of the aorta (with the courtesy of M. Gutberlet, M.D., Leipzig). MR T1-weighted SE sequence (**a**). Stenosis (arrow). Contrast-enhanced MRA (**b**). Stenosis (arrow) and extensive network of collaterals.

▶ **CT and CTA findings**

Findings are identical to MRI ● CT should be used sparingly in children and young patients because of the radiation exposure.

▶ **DSA and cardiac catheterization**
Not indicated as the sole diagnostic study ● May be useful for preoperative pressure measurements ● Used in the setting of interventional therapy.

Clinical Aspects

▶ **Typical presentation**
  - *Adult coarctation:* Often asymptomatic ● Symptoms of arterial hypertension (headache, vertigo, epistaxis) ● Weak leg pulses ● Cardiac failure is present in 65% of patients over 40.
  - *Infantile coarctation:* Severe cardiac failure ● Arterial hypertension ● Cyanosis of the lower half of the body ● Renal failure.

▶ **Therapeutic options**
Surgery or interventional therapy is indicated for a stenosis grade of over 50% or a pressure gradient of over 20 mmHg ● In newborns and infants, the stenosis is usually resected ● Interventional therapy (PTA, stent where indicated) is preferred in older children and adults.

▶ **Course and prognosis**
  - *Adult coarctation:* Left untreated, it leads to severe complications after the age of 40 ● Prognosis improves after treatment even in adults.
  - *Infantile coarctation:* Usually fatal if left untreated ● Prognosis is good after treatment ● Rate of reoccurrence of stenosis after treatment is 3–40% ● Therefore, long-term follow-up with MRI is indicated.

▶ **What does the clinician want to know?**
Grade of stenosis ● Associated malformations ● Hypoplasia of the aortic arch ● Complications (left ventricular hypertrophy or dilation, aortic dissection).

Differential Diagnosis

Pseudocoarctation *of the aorta*	– Hemodynamically insignificant stenosis at the isthmus of the aorta due to elongation and kinking – No collaterals – No difference in blood pressure

Tips and Pitfalls

The severity of the stenosis on color Doppler echocardiography may be overestimated due to aliasing.

Selected References

Abbruzzese PA, Aidala E. Aortic coarctation: an overview. J Cardiovasc Med (Hagerstown) 2007; 8: 123–128

Kramer U et al. [Clinical implication of parameter-optimized 3D-FISP MR angiography (MRA) in children with aortic coarctation: comparison with catheter angiography.] Rofo 2004; 176: 1458–1465 [In German]

Lesko NM et al. The thoracic aorta. In: Grainger RG, Allison DJ (eds.). Diagnostic Radiology. London: Churchill Livingstone; 1997: 859–860

Definition

Synonyms: Aortic arch syndrome, pulseless disease.

▶ **Epidemiology**

Rare in the Caucasian population ● Incidence rate is 0.1–0.3 : 100 000 per year ● Incidence in the Asian population is as much as 10 times higher ● Peak occurrence is at age 20–30 years ● Females are affected about 10 times more often than males.

▶ **Etiology, pathophysiology, pathogenesis**

Systemic vasculitis of the major arteries ● Shows a predilection for the aorta and its major branches as well as the pulmonary arteries ● The florid stage of the disease is characterized by granulomatous inflammation with lymphocytes, macrophages, and giant cells ● Chronic vascular remodeling with scarring ● This leads to stenoses and/or aneurysms.

Imaging Signs

▶ **Modality of choice**

MRI.

▶ **Color Doppler ultrasound findings**

Halo (swelling of the vascular wall) is an early sign of an inflammatory vascular process.

▶ **CT findings**

Active vascular lesion—thickening of the vascular wall after contrast enhancement ● Mural thrombi may be present.

▶ **MRI findings**

Active phase of the disease—thickened vascular wall ● High signal intensity on T2-weighted and postcontrast T1-weighted sequences.

▶ **MRA, CTA, and DSA findings**

Demonstrate late manifestations ● Stenoses ● Occlusions ● Dilations ● Aneurysms.

▶ **FDG-PET**

Full-body screening to demonstrate vasculitis.

Clinical Aspects

▶ **Typical presentation**

Weakness ● Fever ● Night sweats ● Arthralgias and myalgias ● Loss of appetite and weight loss ● Pain in the affected vessels ● Claudication of the extremities, especially the arms ● Impaired vision ● Cerebral infarcts ● Chest and abdominal pain ● Hypertension ● Renal failure ● Laboratory findings include elevated erythrocyte sedimentation rate and C-reactive protein levels.

▶ **Therapeutic options**

Glucocorticoids and immunosuppressives ● Radiologic intervention ● Surgical management.

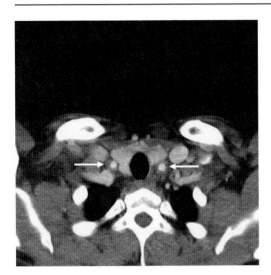

Fig. 4.8 Takayasu arteritis. Axial CT after contrast administration. Halo of soft tissue density (arrows) with increased enhancement of both common carotid arteries.

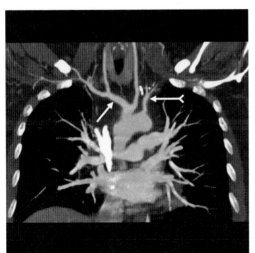

Fig. 4.9 CT after contrast administration, coronal MIP. Findings include wall thickening and irregularities of the lumen along the brachiocephalic trunk (arrow) and left subclavian artery (forked arrow).

▶ **Course and prognosis**
Chronic recurrent course • 5-year mortality is as high as 35% • Cardiac failure • Cerebral or myocardial infarctions • Aneurysm rupture • Renal complications.
▶ **What does the clinician want to know?**
Extent and activity of arterial involvement.

Differential Diagnosis

Giant cell arteritis	– Age over 50 years – Often indistinguishable from Takayasu arteritis in middle-aged patients (45–55 years)
Sarcoidosis	– Hilar and/or mediastinal lymphadenopathy – Changes in the pulmonary parenchyma – Synovitis
Marfan syndrome, Ehlers–Danlos syndrome, and other congenital connective tissue disorders	– The typical manifestations do not include stenoses of the major arteries – No systemic symptoms
Atherosclerosis	– Usually affects older patients – Predilection for the lower extremity arteries and the abdominal aorta
Infectious causes	– Stenosis of the origin of the supraaortic artery is not common

Tips and Pitfalls

There are no pathognomonic radiologic or serologic findings; the diagnosis is made on the basis of characteristic clinical manifestations in combination with corresponding vascular changes on imaging studies.

Selected References

Fritz J et al. [Current imaging in Takayasu arteritis.] Rofo 2005; 177: 1467–1472 [In German]

Gotway MB et al. Imaging findings in Takayasu's arteritis. AJR Am J Roentgenol 2005; 184: 1945–1950

Kissin EY, Merkel PA. Diagnostic imaging in Takayasu arteritis. Curr Opin Rheumatol 2004; 16: 31–37

Sueyashi E et al. MRI of Takayasu's arteritis: typical appearances and complications. AJR Am J Roentgenol 2006; 187: W569–W575

Definition

▶ **Epidemiology**
Prevalence in autopsy material is 1.1–1.5% • Incidence rate is 3 : 100000 yearly •
In emergency rooms about one acute aortic syndrome occurs per 80–300 cases
of acute coronary syndrome • It is the thirteenth most common cause of death in
people over 65 years • In the past 10 years, deaths attributable to acute aortic
syndrome have doubled, a fact that probably reflects improvements in diagnostic imaging.

▶ **Etiology, pathophysiology, pathogenesis**
The term has only recently entered published literature • It encompasses a range
of nontraumatic acute life-threatening disorders of the thoracic aorta:
  – Aortic dissection
  – Intramural hematoma
  – Penetrating aortic ulcer
  – Ruptured aneurysm.
  – These entities are clinically indistinguishable or at best poorly distinguish-
    able • Diagnosis is made by imaging studies • The most important causes
    are atherosclerosis and arterial hypertension • Other causes are listed under
    the individual diagnoses.

Imaging Signs

▶ **Modality of choice**
CTA, including CT coronary imaging and pulmonary CTA (chest pain protocol)
where applicable.

▶ **Findings**
The imaging findings depend on the specific disorder—see relevant sections.

Clinical Aspects

▶ **Typical presentation**
Acute stabbing chest or back pain • Excruciating pain • Pain may radiate into the
neck or abdomen • Easily mistaken for angina pectoris • There may be a pulse
and blood pressure difference between the upper and lower extremities.

▶ **Therapeutic options**
The treatment varies according to the specific disorders—see relevant sections.

▶ **Course and prognosis**
The mortality rate for untreated cases is high (about 80%); death usually occurs
because of aortic rupture • For further information about course and prognosis,
see the specific disorders.

▶ **What does the clinician want to know?**
Rapid recognition of the cause of the acute chest pain (see the specific disorders).

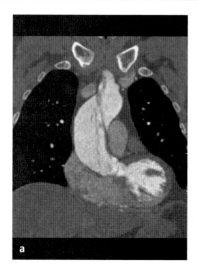 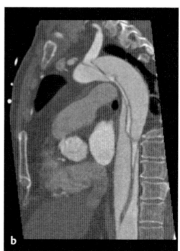

Fig. 4.10 a, b Acute dissection of the ascending and descending aorta (type A, Stanford classification). CTA.

Differential Diagnosis

Acute coronary syndrome	– Stenosis and/or occlusion of coronary arteries
Pulmonary artery embolism	– Contrast filling defects in pulmonary arteries
Acute abdomen	– Extensive list of causes, many of which can be revealed using CT

Tips and Pitfalls

Failure to visualize the abdominal aorta.

Selected References

von Kodolitsch Y et al. [The acute aortic syndrome.] Dtsch Arztebl 2003; 100: A326–333 [In German]

Manghat NE et al. Multi-detector row computed tomography: imaging in acute aortic syndrome. Clin Radiol 2005; 60: 1256–1267

Romano L et al. Multidetector-row CT evaluation of nontraumatic acute thoracic aortic syndromes. Radiol Med (Torino) 2007; 112: 1–20

Schmidt M et al. [Imaging of acute aortic syndromes.] Rofo 2007; 179: 551–554 [In German]

Vilacosta I, Roman JA. Acute aortic syndrome. Heart 2001; 85: 365–368

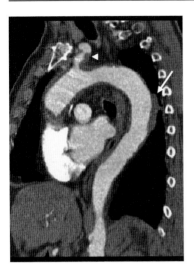

Fig. 4.11 Intramural hematoma (arrow) of the descending aorta. CTA. Additional findings include uncalcified plaques in the aortic arch and at the origin of the left subclavian artery (arrowhead). In contrast with the plaques, the hematoma primarily projects outward.

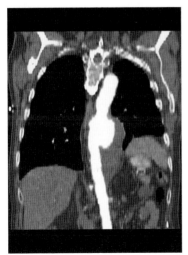

Fig. 4.12 Ruptured aortic aneurysm. CTA.

Definition

▶ **Epidemiology**

Incidence is unknown • As familiarity with the disorder increases, it is diagnosed more often • Occurs in 5–10% of patients with acute aortic syndrome • Males are affected more often than females.

▶ **Etiology, pathophysiology, pathogenesis**

Atherosclerotic ulcer that penetrates into the media through the elastica interna • There it usually causes a hematoma • Can be regarded as a forme fruste of a dissection in which hard atherosclerotic plaques prevent the longitudinal progression of the dissection • Size varies from a few millimeters to up to 2.5 cm (transverse diameter and depth) • Most often occurs in the descending aorta • Risk factors include advanced atherosclerosis and arterial hypertension • Aortic dissection, intramural aortic hematoma, and penetrating aortic ulcer are closely related disorders and are probably manifestations of a continuous disease spectrum.

Imaging Signs

▶ **Modality of choice**

CT and CTA • MRI and MRA.

▶ **Transesophageal echocardiography findings**

Localized, craterlike expansion of the lumen into the wall of the aorta • Usually there are severe, generalized atherosclerotic changes in the aortic wall.

▶ **CT and CTA findings**

Unenhanced scans in acute or subacute disease may show a hyperdense hematoma of the aortic wall • Contrast-enhanced images show localized, craterlike expansion of the lumen into the aortic wall • The wall around the ulcer is thickened and enhances • Usually there are severe, generalized atherosclerotic changes in the aortic wall.

▶ **MRI and MRA findings**

T1-weighted SE sequences in acute or subacute disease show a hyperintense hematoma • Otherwise findings are identical to contrast CT • The advantage of MRI is that it can distinguish hematoma from atherosclerotic plaque • Less suitable for acute cases.

▶ **DSA findings**

Focal expansion of the lumen into the aortic wall • Several oblique projections may be required to detect smaller ulcers • Obsolete for diagnostic purposes • Performed in the setting of endovascular therapy.

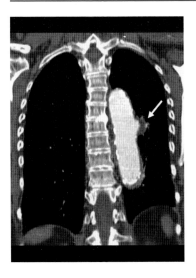

Fig. 4.13 Penetrating ulcer of the descending aorta. CTA. Caplike intramural hematoma (arrow).

Clinical Aspects

▶ **Typical presentation**
  Severe acute chest pain radiating into the back ● Often asymptomatic ● May be an incidental finding.

▶ **Therapeutic options**
  Initially conservative antihypertensive therapy is indicated ● Where complications occur (persistent pain, enlargement, perforation, embolization), stent grafting or surgery is indicated.

▶ **Course and prognosis**
  Prognosis is good for stable forms under conservative treatment ● Some ulcers are unstable and progress to dissection, aneurysm, pseudoaneurysm, or rupture.

▶ **What does the clinician want to know?**
  Location ● Size, especially over time ● Complications (dissection, aneurysm, rupture).

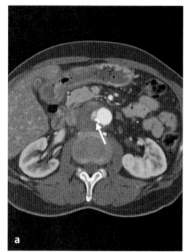

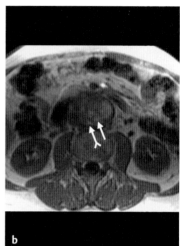

Fig. 4.14 a–c Penetrating ulcer (arrow) of the abdominal aorta with a large accompanying hematoma. **a** CTA. **b** Axial T1-weighted MR image shows hyperintense areas (forked arrow) within the hematoma. **c** Coronal contrast-enhanced MRA.

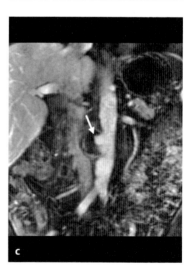

Differential Diagnosis

Aortic dissection	– More extensive than an aortic ulcer – Two distinct lumina – Atherosclerosis tends to be less severe (but seamless transition from ulcer to dissection)
Thrombosed dissection	– Usually more extensive than an aortic ulcer – Can be a sequela of an aortic ulcer
Intramural hematoma	– No ulcer crater – Intima is intact
Aortic aneurysm with thrombus along the aortic wall	– More extensive than an aortic ulcer – Typical aneurysm form
Ulcerated atherosclerotic plaques	– Less circumscribed – Disseminated calcifications – Hypointense on T1-weighted images

Tips and Pitfalls

Failure to detect the disorder due to lack of familiarity with it • Neglecting to obtain an unenhanced CT scan.

Selected References

Hayashi H et al. Penetrating atherosclerotic ulcer of the aorta: imaging features and disease concept. RadioGraphics 2000; 20: 995–1005

Manghat NE et al. Multi-detector row computed tomography: imaging in acute aortic syndrome. Clin Radiol 2005; 60: 1256–1267

Stanson AW et al. Penetrating atherosclerotic ulcers of the thoracic aorta: natural history and clinicopathologic correlations. Ann Vasc Surg 1986; 1: 15–23

Sundt TM. Intramural hematoma and penetrating atherosclerotic ulcer of the aorta. Ann Thorac Surg 2007; 83: S835–841

Definition

▸ **Epidemiology**
Occurs in 5–20% of patients with acute aortic syndrome.

▸ **Etiology, pathophysiology, pathogenesis**
Usually circumscribed hemorrhage in the media of the aortic wall ● Most often hemorrhage from the vasa vasorum with an intact intima and no communication with the aortic lumen ● May also be caused by a penetrating aortic ulcer ● Stanford classification is used as with aortic dissection ● Aortic dissection, intramural aortic hematoma, and penetrating aortic ulcer are closely related disorders and are probably manifestations of a continuous disease spectrum.

Imaging Signs

▸ **Modality of choice**
CT and CTA ● MRI and MRA.

▸ **Transesophageal echocardiography**
Localized, thrombuslike swelling of the wall ● Crescentic ● Hypoechoic ● Intimal calcifications are separated from the rest of the wall by the hematoma ● Lumen is smooth without any intimal defect ● A disadvantage is that the modality does not visualize the entire aorta.

▸ **CT and CTA findings**
Modality of choice for planning intervention ● Unenhanced scans in acute or subacute disease show a hyperdense hematoma of the aortic wall ● Contrast sequences show a localized, crescentic, thrombuslike swelling of the wall ● Any intimal calcifications are separated from the rest of the wall by the hematoma ● Lumen is smooth without any intimal defect ● Pulsation artifacts in the ascending aorta can be suppressed by ECG gating.

▸ **MRI and MRA findings**
Modality of choice for demonstrating recurrent hemorrhage ● T1-weighted SE sequences in acute or subacute disease show a hyperintense hematoma ● This allows estimation of the age of the lesion ● Otherwise findings are identical to contrast CT ● Less suitable for acute cases.

▸ **DSA findings**
Findings are normal in 85% of all cases.

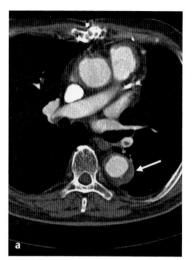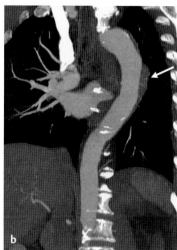

Fig. 4.15 a, b Intramural hematoma of the aorta. CTA, axial (**a**) and coronal (**b**). Circumscribed intramural hematoma (arrow) of the descending aorta (type B). Incidental findings include pulmonary artery embolism (**a**).

Clinical Aspects

▶ **Typical presentation**
Severe acute chest pain radiating into the back.

▶ **Therapeutic options**
Type A is treated by surgical replacement of the ascending aorta • Type B is treated conservatively by antihypertensive therapy • Where complications occur, surgery or stent grafting is indicated.

▶ **Course and prognosis**
  – *Type A:* In 80% of all cases, a type A dissection occurs in the course of the disease • Early mortality is 42% • Surgical treatment improves the prognosis.
  – *Type B:* Often resolves with no sequelae • Dissection or aneurysm may occur • Early mortality is 8%.

▶ **What does the clinician want to know?**
Position and type of hematoma • Size • Acuity, especially where recurrent hemorrhage is suspected • Complications (dissection, aneurysm).

Differential Diagnosis

Thrombosed dissection	– Intimal defect is present but in the presence of thrombosis, it is often not clearly visualized – Usually more extensive than an intramural hematoma – Sometimes indistinguishable from intramural hematoma
Penetrating aortic ulcer	– Short focal defect in the intima and media with expansion of the lumen into the aortic wall – Often associated with a secondary aortic wall hematoma
Aortic aneurysm with thrombus along the aortic wall	– Typical aneurysm form – Usually there are significant irregularities of the lumen
Atherosclerotic plaques	– Less circumscribed – Disseminated calcifications – Significant irregularities of the lumen

Tips and Pitfalls

Failure to detect the lesion because of lack of familiarity with it ● Neglecting to obtain an unenhanced CT scan.

Selected References

Dieckmann C et al. [Intramural hemorrhage of the thoracic aorta.] Rofo 1998; 169: 370–377 [In German]

Manghat NE et al. Multi-detector row computed tomography: imaging in acute aortic syndrome. Clin Radiol 2005; 60: 1256–1267

Murray JG et al. Intramural hematoma of the thoracic aorta: MR image findings and their prognostic implications. Radiology 1997; 204: 349–355

Sundt TM. Intramural hematoma and penetrating atherosclerotic ulcer of the aorta. Ann Thorac Surg 2007; 83: S835–841; discussion S846–850

Definition

▶ **Epidemiology**

Incidence rate is 2–5 : 100 000 per year ● Males are affected about twice as often as females ● Peak age is 40–80 years.

▶ **Etiology, pathophysiology, pathogenesis**

Blood enters the media through a proximal tear in the intima, opening a second "false" lumen between the middle and outer thirds of the media (the path of least resistance) ● This second lumen then propagates distally, often eventually merging with the true lumen (reentry point) ● The most common cause is atherosclerosis with chronic arterial hypertension ● Less common causes include trauma, Marfan syndrome, bicuspid aortic valve, coarctation of the aorta, arteritis, and pregnancy ● Aortic dissection, intramural aortic hematoma, and penetrating aortic ulcer are closely related disorders and are probably manifestations of a continuous disease spectrum.

Imaging Signs

▶ **Modality of choice**

CTA.

▶ **Transesophageal echocardiography findings**

Dilated aorta ● Intimal flap with blood flow in the true and false lumens ● The advantage is that complications (pericardial tamponade, coronary artery involvement, and aortic insufficiency) are readily identifiable ● Disadvantages are that involvement of the major aortic branches (carotids and renal arteries), a reentry point distal to the diaphragm, and signs of imminent rupture can only be evaluated to a limited extent.

▶ **CTA findings**

Dilated aorta ● Intimal flap ● The true lumen is usually the smaller lumen with more pronounced enhancement on early scans ● The false lumen is larger and enhances later ● There may be fine strands of tissue bridging the false lumen ("cobwebs") ● The false lumen may be thrombosed ● The advantage of CT is that it visualizes all affected arteries and organs ● Cardiac complications can also be readily visualized with multislice CT ● Mediastinal hematoma and hemothorax are signs of imminent or acute rupture ● Modality of choice for planning intervention ● Pulsation artifacts in the ascending aorta can be suppressed by ECG gating.

▶ **MRA and MRI findings**

Findings are identical to CTA ● Less suitable for acute cases ● Indicated for follow-up of chronic dissections ● Cardiac function can be readily evaluated.

▶ **DSA findings**

Dilated aorta ● Intimal flap ● The true lumen is usually the smaller lumen and fills earlier ● The false lumen is larger and fills later ● Has largely fallen out of favor as a diagnostic modality ● Only performed in the setting of endovascular therapy.

Fig. 4.16 Stanford classification of aortic dissection (now generally used as it is based on therapeutic relevance): *Type A*—dissection involving the ascending aorta; *Type B*—dissection not involving the ascending aorta. DeBakey classification (now only rarely used): *Type I*—beginning in the ascending aorta and continuing in the aortic arch and descending aorta; *Type II*—affects only the ascending aorta; *Type III*—affects only the descending aorta.

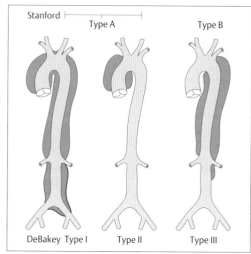

Clinical Aspects

▶ **Typical presentation**
Severe acute chest pain radiating into the back • Asymptomatic in about 25% of all cases • Shock • Neurologic deficits • Hypertensive crisis (renal artery involvement) • Bowel ischemia • Ischemia in the lower extremities • Type A is also associated with pericardial tamponade, aortic insufficiency, and myocardial infarction (coronary artery involvement).

▶ **Therapeutic options**
– *Type A* (Stanford classification): Treated with immediate surgical replacement of the ascending aorta • Aortic valve replacement may be indicated.
– *Type B* (Stanford classification): Treated conservatively by antihypertensive therapy in uncomplicated cases • Complicated cases (severe ischemia, imminent rupture) are treated by stent graft and endovascular fenestration where indicated.

▶ **Course and prognosis**
In type A, mortality is 1% per hour until surgery • In type B, the 5-year survival rate is 60%.

▶ **What does the clinician want to know?**
Type and extent of dissection • Perfusion or thrombosis of the false lumen • Cardiac complications • Involvement of aortic branches with ischemia • Acute risk of rupture • Measurement of the size of the aorta for selection of a stent.

Differential Diagnosis

Intramural hematoma	– Crescentic thickening of the aortic wall
	– No perfused false lumen

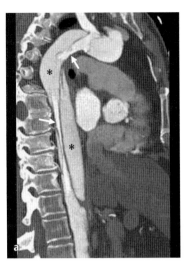 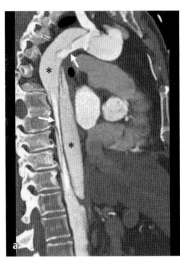

Fig. 4.17 a, b   Type A aortic dissection (Stanford classification). CT angiography. Small compressed true lumen with increased enhancement (arrows). Large peripheral false lumen with less enhancement (asterisk).

	– Intima is intact
	– Sometimes indistinguishable from dissection with thrombosed false lumen
Traumatic aortic rupture	– Defect in the aortic wall
	– Mediastinal hematoma
	– No typical intimal flap
Penetrating aortic ulcer	– Short focal defect in the intima and media with expansion of the lumen into the aortic wall
	– No intimal flap
Thoracic aortic aneurysm	– Enlarged aorta with thrombus along the aortic wall
	– No intimal flap, no false lumen

Tips and Pitfalls

Pulsation artifacts in the ascending aorta can be confused with an intimal flap on CT.

Selected References

Kapustin AJ, Litt HI. Diagnostic imaging for aortic dissection. Semin Thorac Cardiovasc Surg 2005; 17: 214–223

O'Gara P. Aortic dissection: Pathophysiology, clinical evaluation, and medical management. In: Creager MA et al. (eds). Vascular Medicine: A Companion to Braunwald's Heart Disease. Philadelphia: Saunders; 2006

Sbarzaglia P et al. Interventional techniques in the treatment of aortic dissection. Radiol Med (Torino) 2006; 111: 585–596

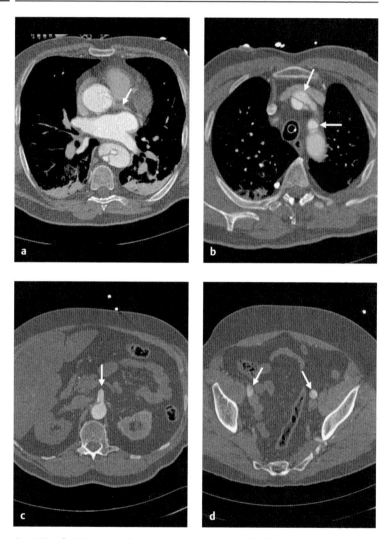

Fig. 4.18 a–d CT angiography (same patient as in Fig. 4.**17**). The dissection extends to the following vessels: the main trunk of the left coronary artery (arrow) with occlusion of the artery (**a**) and myocardial infarction; the supraaortic branches (**b**, arrows); the superior mesenteric artery (**c**, arrow); and both iliac arteries (**d**, arrows).

Definition

▶ **Epidemiology**
Occurs in 3 of 1000 patients with blunt chest trauma.

▶ **Etiology, pathophysiology, pathogenesis**
Shear forces in sudden deceleration from high speeds (usually motor vehicle accidents) cause injury to the aortic wall ● Injury typically occurs (in 90% of cases) at the aortic isthmus (concavity) at the junction between the relatively flexible aortic arch and the fixed descending aorta ● Complete ruptures (occurring in 80–90% of cases) cause immediate death due to massive blood loss ● In incomplete ruptures, the intact adventitia initially prevents massive bleeding ● Severe associated injuries are present in 90% of patients.

Imaging Signs

▶ **Modality of choice**
CTA as part of whole-body CT in patients with multiple trauma.

▶ **Standard supine chest radiograph findings**
Irregular contour of the aorta ● Widening of the mediastinum (often difficult to evaluate in the supine patient) ● Trachea is displaced to the right, and gastric tube may be as well ● Left main bronchus is displaced caudally ● Findings usually include hemothorax on the left side ● Hematoma of the left apical parietal pleura ("apical pleural cap") ● Standard chest radiograph shows abnormal findings in 93% of patients.

▶ **Transesophageal echocardiography findings**
Pseudoaneurysm of the aorta with irregular contour of the aortic wall ● Flap of variable thickness ● Flap consists of intima or intima and media ● Turbulent flow on color Doppler ● Mediastinal hematoma (usually due to tearing of small mediastinal veins) ● Very precise but invasive modality ● Usually used to supplement CTA in uncertain cases.

▶ **CTA findings**
Pseudoaneurysm of the aorta with irregular contour of the aortic wall ● Flap of variable thickness ● Mediastinal hematoma ● Hemothorax on the left side ● Pulsation artifacts in the ascending aorta can be suppressed by ECG gating.

▶ **DSA findings**
Pseudoaneurysm of the aorta with irregular contour of the aortic wall ● Flap of variable thickness ● Now obsolete for diagnostic purposes ● Performed in the setting of endovascular therapy.

Fig. 4.19 a, b Incomplete traumatic aortic rupture at the typical site. Axial (**a**) and sagittal (**b**) CTA. Irregular aortic wall, pseudoaneurysm, flap (arrows), and mediastinal hematoma (asterisks). Trachea and gastric tube are displaced to the right.

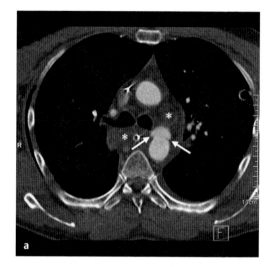

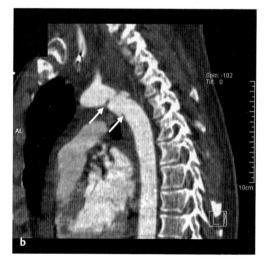

Clinical Aspects

▶ **Typical presentation**
Patients with multiple trauma from severe deceleration (such as motor vehicle accidents or falls from a great height) ● External chest injuries ● Hypovolemic shock may occur.

▶ **Therapeutic options**
Stent graft ● Surgery.

▶ **Course and prognosis**
There is no chance of survival with a complete rupture occurring at the time of the injury ● In untreated incomplete rupture, 80% of patients die within 24 hours and 98% within 10 weeks ● With treatment, 60–70% of patients survive ● Associated injuries increase the mortality rate.

▶ **What does the clinician want to know?**
Location of the rupture ● Size of the mediastinal hematoma ● Associated injuries ● Measurement of the size of the aorta for selection of the stent.

Differential Diagnosis

Preexisting thoracic aortic aneurysm or chronic aortic dissection in trauma patients	– Chronic thrombus along the aortic wall – No mediastinal hematoma – Significant calcifications

Tips and Pitfalls

Pulsation artifacts in the ascending aorta can be confused with an intimal flap on CT ● In young adults, residual thymic tissue may be confused with a mediastinal hematoma.

Selected References

Albrecht T et al. [The role of whole body spiral CT in the primary work-up of polytrauma patients—comparison with conventional radiography and abdominal sonography.] Rofo 2004; 176: 1142–1150 [In German]

Balm R, Hoornweg LL. Traumatic aortic ruptures. J Cardiovasc Surg (Torino) 2005; 46: 101–105

Bohndorf K et al. [Diagnosis of posttraumatic ruptures of the thoracic aorta using chest x-ray and angiography.] Rofo 1984; 140: 515–519

Manghat NE et al. Multi-detector row computed tomography: imaging in acute aortic syndrome. Clin Radiol 2005; 60: 1256–1267

Vignon P et al. Role of transesophageal echocardiography in the diagnosis and management of traumatic aortic disruption. Circulation 1995; 92: 2959–2968

Definition
....

▶ **Epidemiology**
Occurs significantly less often than abdominal aortic aneurysm • Prevalence is
4.5 : 100 000 • Incidence in the Western world has decreased in recent decades
as control of syphilis has improved • Males are affected three times more often
than females.

▶ **Etiology, pathophysiology, pathogenesis**
Circumscribed fusiform (80% of cases) or saccular dilation of the thoracic aorta
to over 150% of normal size • *Location:* 60% occur in the ascending aorta (10% of
these in aortic arch), 40% in the descending aorta (10% of these in abdominal aorta), • Most common causes include cystic medial necrosis (in the ascending aorta) and atherosclerosis (descending aorta) with or without arterial hypertension • Rare causes include aortic defects, posttraumatic conditions (pseudoaneurysm), cystic medial necrosis, syphilis, arteritis, and Marfan syndrome.

Imaging Signs
....

▶ **Modality of choice**
CTA.

▶ **Standard chest radiograph findings**
Widening of the mediastinum • Enlargement or widening of the aortic arch and
aortic silhouette • Shell-like calcifications • Tracheal deviation.

▶ **Transesophageal echocardiography findings**
Circumscribed fusiform or saccular dilation of the aorta • Thrombus along the
aortic wall can be readily distinguished from the lumen on color Doppler studies • The advantage is that associated cardiac disorders, especially aortic valve
defects, can be readily evaluated • The disadvantage is that the exact position
of the supraaortic branches cannot be evaluated.

▶ **CTA findings**
Circumscribed fusiform or saccular dilation of the aorta • Thrombus along the
aortic wall • Crescentic calcification of the aneurysmal wall • Findings may include left ventricular dilation and/or hypertrophy • The advantage is that the
spacial relationship of the supra-aortic branches to the aneurysm can be clearly
evaluated on multiplanar reconstructions • Modality of choice for planning a
stent graft.

▶ **MRA and MRI findings**
Findings are identical to CTA • Lumen and thrombus may be indistinguishable
without contrast material • Calcifications along the aortic wall are not usually
visible.

▶ **DSA findings**
Dilation of the aorta is usually considerably less than the actual size of the aneurysm as only the lumen is visualized but not the thrombus • The origins of the
intercostal arteries are occluded • Obsolete for diagnostic purposes • Performed
in the setting of endovascular therapy.

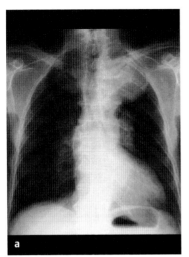 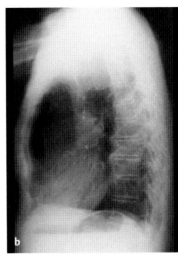

Fig. 4.20 a, b Thoracic aortic aneurysm. Radiographs of the chest in two planes. Large thoracic aneurysm arising from the aortic arch.

Table 4.1 Diagnostic values

Segment of vessel	Normal outer diameter	Aneurysm
Ascending aorta	≤ 3 cm	≥ 5 cm
Descending aorta	≤ 2.5 cm	≥ 4 cm

Clinical Aspects

▶ **Typical presentation**

From 25 % to 50 % of cases are asymptomatic • Symptoms usually occur only in large aneurysms • Retrosternal pain • Back pain • Dysphagia • Dyspnea • Upper venous congestion in the superior blood vessels • Hoarseness (recurrent nerve palsy).

▶ **Therapeutic options**

Surgery in the ascending aorta and aortic arch • Stent graft or surgery in the descending aorta • Surgery or endovascular therapy are indicated for diameters greater than or equal to 6 cm and in symptomatic cases where the diameter increases 1 cm per year.

▶ **Course and prognosis**

Slowly increases in size, thus increasing the risk of rupture • Annual rupture rate: < 5 cm: 2 %; 5–5.9 cm: 3 %; ≥ 6 cm: 7 % • Prognosis is good after successful therapy.

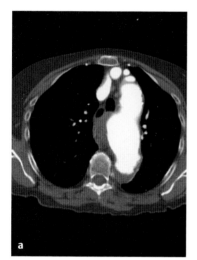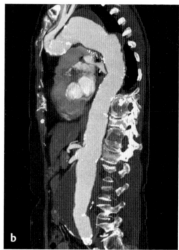

Fig. 4.21 a, b   Thoracoabdominal aortic aneurysm. CTA, axial image (**a**) and parasagittal multiplanar reconstruction along the aorta (**b**). The aneurysm begins distal to the isthmus of the aorta.

► **What does the clinician want to know?**

Size and position of the aneurysm ● Signs of imminent rupture ("crescent sign": hyperdense thrombus on unenhanced CT scans, contrast-filled tears in the thrombus) or signs of a rupture that has already occurred (see "Ruptured thoracic aneurysm") ● Condition of other major arteries (further aneurysms, stenoses) ● Measurement of the size of the aorta for selection of stent.

Differential Diagnosis

Intramural hematoma	– Crescentic thickening of the aortic wall with expansion of the outer diameter of the aorta; lumen width remains normal
	– There may be intimal calcification between the lumen and hematoma (calcification of the aortic wall is peripheral to the thrombus in aneurysms)
Penetrating aortic ulcer	– Short focal defect in the intima and media with expansion of the lumen into the aortic wall
	– Usually a small localized hematoma
	– Lumen width remains normal
Pseudoaneurysm	– Surrounded only by adventitia and connective tissue
	– Often indistinguishable on imaging studies
	– Usually posttraumatic or iatrogenic; history is therefore the most important criterion

Tips and Pitfalls

Failure to visualize the abdominal aorta • Size measurement must be made on the basis of outer diameter.

Selected References

Black JH 3rd, Cambria RP. Current results of open surgical repair of descending thoracic aortic aneurysms. J Vasc Surg 2006; 43 Suppl A: A6–11

Isselbacher EM. Thoracic and abdominal aortic aneurysms. Circulation 2005; 111: 816–828

Kougias P et al. Endovascular management of thoracic aortic aneurysms. Preoperative imaging and device sizing. J Vasc Surg 2006; 43 Suppl A: A48–52

Nataf P, Lansac E. Dilation of the thoracic aorta: medical and surgical management. Heart 2006; 92: 1345–1352

Definition

▶ **Epidemiology**
Relative frequency among all aneurysms is 0.8–3.3%.

▶ **Etiology, pathophysiology, pathogenesis**
Aneurysm occurs as a result of microbial infection ● Preexisting aneurysms rarely become infected ● Most common pathogens are staphylococci and salmonellae ● Infection may be hematogenous (pneumonia or sepsis), lymphatic (tuberculous aortitis), by direct spread (suppurative pericarditis, osteomyelitis), or posttraumatic and/or iatrogenic ● The suprarenal segments of the aorta are involved in two-thirds of cases.

Imaging Signs

▶ **Modality of choice**
CTA.

▶ **CTA findings**
Typically occurs as a saccular aneurysm with a lobulated contour ● Perianeurysmal fluid retention in fatty tissue and/or fluid accumulation ● Gas inclusions may be present ● Rapid expansion.

▶ **MRI findings**
T1-weighted sequences, with contrast material, are especially suitable for visualizing perianeurysmal inflammatory reactions.

Clinical Aspects

▶ **Typical presentation**
Nonspecific generalized symptoms ● Local inflammatory reactions (fever, pain) ● Blood cultures are positive in about 75% of cases.

▶ **Therapeutic options**
Intravenous antibiotic therapy ● Emergency surgery ● Lifelong antibiotic prophylaxis.

▶ **Course and prognosis**
Rapid increase in size (develops within a few days) ● High risk of rupture (at the time of surgery more than half of all aneurysms have already ruptured) ● Mortality is 16–40%.

▶ **What does the clinician want to know?**
Signs of infectious etiology of the aneurysm ● Focus of infection ● Rupture.

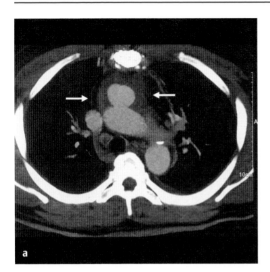

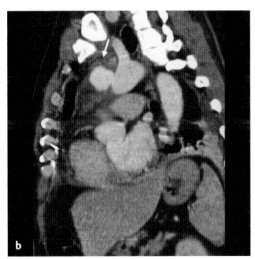

Fig. 4.22 a, b Infectious aneurysm of the ascending aorta after heart surgery. CT after contrast administration. Axial MIP (**a**) and sagittal reconstruction (**b**). The aneurysm is surrounded by a ring of connective tissue with inflammatory infiltrate (arrows) that shows increased enhancement.

Differential Diagnosis

Atherosclerotic aneurysm	– Preexisting vascular pathology with vascular calcifications
	– Saccular and fusiform
	– Slowly increases in size
Inflammatory aneurysm	– Occurs in the infrarenal aorta and pelvic arteries
	– Retroperitoneal fibrosis, detectable on contrast-enhanced CT as perianeurysmal hyperdensity with medial displacement of the ureters and occasionally stenosis of the vena cava.

Tips and Pitfalls

Misinterpreting the cause of the aneurysm.

Selected References

Macedo TA et al. Infected aortic aneurysms: imaging findings. Radiology 2004; 231: 250–257

Malouf JF et al. Mycotic aneurysms of the thoracic aorta: A diagnostic challenge. Am J Med 2003; 115: 489–496

Welborn MB, Valentine RJ. Vascular infection. In: Creager MA et al. (eds.). Vascular Medicine: A Companion to Braunwald's Heart Disease. Philadelphia: Saunders; 2006

Definition

▶ **Epidemiology**
Occurs significantly less often than a ruptured abdominal aortic aneurysm • The annual rupture rate of thoracic aortic aneurysms depends on their diameter: < 5 cm: 2 %; 5–5.9 cm: 3 %; ≥ 6 cm: 7 %.

▶ **Etiology, pathophysiology, pathogenesis**
Preexisting aneurysm or pseudoaneurysm of the thoracic aorta • Additional risk factors include arterial hypertension, chronic lung infection, female sex, and smoking • There is progressive disintegration of the aortic wall • The lesion begins as a hemorrhage into a thrombus and the aortic wall • This develops into a small leak with a mediastinal hematoma • Finally a complete rupture develops • Rupture may occur into the esophagus, pleural space, or pericardium.

Imaging Signs

▶ **Modality of choice**
CTA.

▶ **Standard chest radiograph findings**
Widening of the mediastinum • Widening, blurring, or loss of contour of the aorta • The trachea is displaced to the right, and the gastric tube may be as well • Left main bronchus is displaced caudally • Findings usually include hemothorax on the left side • Hematoma of the left apical parietal pleura ("apical pleural cap") • The standard chest radiograph shows low sensitivity in detecting ruptures.

▶ **Transesophageal echocardiography findings**
Aneurysm • Mediastinal hematoma is often difficult to detect.

▶ **CTA findings**
Aneurysm • Diagnostic is the visualization of a mediastinal hematoma with CT • Findings usually include hemothorax on the left side • There may be contrast extravasation • Hemopericardium • Blood or contrast in the esophagus • The modality has the advantages of being quick (which is decisive), comprehensive, (visualizing the entire aorta and major branches), and sensitive.
Rapidly increasing size is a sign of imminent rupture • Increased size of lumen relative to thrombus • Crescent of calcification is interrupted • "Crescent sign" (originally described on unenhanced CT scans—a hyperdense crescent in the thrombus consistent with acute hemorrhage) • Contrast crescent visualized within the thrombus on CTA.

▶ **MRA and DSA**
Contraindicated in acute cases due to the time required for the study.

Fig. 4.23 a, b   Ruptured thoracic aortic aneurysm. CTA. Rupture of the thoracic aortic aneurysm (arrow) has produced an extensive mediastinal hematoma (asterisk). Incidental findings include a gastric tube (triangle).

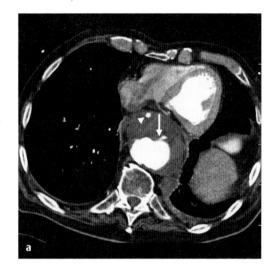

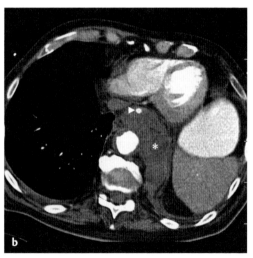

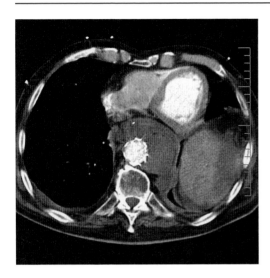

Fig. 4.24 Same patient as in **Fig. 4.23** after placement of a stent graft.

Clinical Aspects

▶ **Typical presentation**

Acute stabbing chest or back pain • Excruciating pain • Hypovolemic shock • There may a difference in the pulse and blood pressure between the upper and lower extremities.

▶ **Therapeutic options**

Immediate surgery • Acute aneurysms of the descending aorta are also increasingly treated with stent graft.

▶ **Course and prognosis**

High mortality, especially in complete rupture or involvement of the ascending aorta • Many patients fail to reach the operating room in time • High perioperative morbidity (including paraplegia and acute renal failure) and mortality (about 25%) • Less with endovascular therapy.

▶ **What does the clinician want to know?**

Acute contrast extravasation • Size of the hematoma • Position and size of the aneurysm • Involvement of supraaortic branches • Aortic insufficiency • Hemopericardium • Measurement of the size of the aorta for selection of stent.

Differential Diagnosis

Ruptured penetrating aortic ulcer	– Short focal defect in the intima and media with expansion of the lumen into the aortic wall
	– Hematoma in the aortic wall and mediastinum
	– Note: Aortic aneurysm and penetrating aortic ulcer often occur simultaneously

Tips and Pitfalls

Delay in obtaining diagnostic imaging studies ● Failure to visualize the abdominal aorta ● *Caution:* A rapid, large contrast bolus can increase blood pressure and stroke volume, which may lead to a fatal complete rupture.

Selected References

Black JH 3rd, Cambria RP. Current results of open surgical repair of descending thoracic aortic aneurysms. J Vasc Surg 2006; 43 Suppl A: A6–11

Manghat NE et al. Multi-detector row computed tomography: imaging in acute aortic syndrome. Clin Radiol 2005; 60: 1256–1267

Nataf P, Lansac E. Dilation of the thoracic aorta: Medical and surgical management. Heart 2006; 92: 1345–1352

Definition

▶ **Epidemiology**
Annual incidence rate of venous thromboembolism (deep venous thrombosis and pulmonary embolism) is about 1 : 1000.

▶ **Etiology, pathophysiology, pathogenesis**
In over 90% of cases, the disorder is a complication of deep venous thrombosis in the pelvis or lower extremity ● For risk factors, see the section "Venous Thrombosis in the Pelvis and Lower Extremity" ● Hemodynamic derangement ● Reduction in right and left ventricular output ● Impaired gas exchange in the lungs.

Imaging Signs

▶ **Modality of choice**
CTA.

▶ **Chest ultrasound findings**
Only indicated in exceptional cases such as adverse reaction to contrast medium, renal failure, and pregnancy ● Typical findings include round to triangular pleural hypoechoic areas exceeding 5 mm in diameter.

▶ **Echocardiography findings**
Used in the presence of confirmed pulmonary embolism to estimate risk by measuring right ventricular pressure and dysfunction.

▶ **Ventilation/perfusion nuclear medicine imaging**
A positive finding (mismatch) has high predictive value ● However, half of all examinations produce indeterminate findings.

▶ **Standard chest radiograph findings**
Findings are often normal or include only discrete abnormalities ● Classic findings such as local oligemia (Westermark sign), a ballooned hilar artery with an abrupt change in caliber (knuckle sign), and a peripheral wedge-shaped density (Hampton hump) are rare.

▶ **CTA findings**
Combined CT angiography and pelvic CT venography can provide additional information about the source of the embolus ● Filling defects in pulmonary arteries ● Vascular dilation.

▶ **MRA findings**
Findings are similar to CT.

▶ **Pulmonary angiography**
Now only rarely indicated.

Fig. 4.25 Pulmonary embolism. CTA. Thromboembolic filling defects in the main pulmonary arteries and their branches.

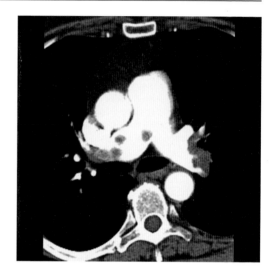

Fig. 4.26 CT venography (same patient as in **Fig. 4.25**). Acute thrombosis of the right internal iliac vein (arrow).

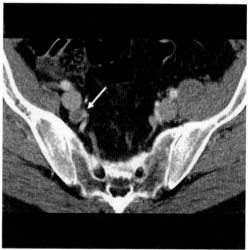

Clinical Aspects

▸ **Typical presentation**
Acute dyspnea ● Chest pain ● Syncope ● Hemoptysis ● Positive D-dimer test.

▸ **Therapeutic options**
– *Risk group I* (stable hemodynamics without right ventricular dysfunction): Anticoagulation as in deep venous thrombosis.
– *Risk group II* (stable hemodynamics with right ventricular dysfunction): Anticoagulation ● Systemic thrombolysis may be indicated.
– *Risk groups III and IV* (in shock or requiring resuscitation): Systemic thrombolysis in addition to anticoagulation with unfractionated heparin ● An alternative is mechanical recanalization.
– Secondary prophylaxis with vitamin K antagonists.

▸ **Course and prognosis**
Up to 90% of deaths occur within 1–2 hours of the onset of symptoms ● Proper anticoagulation reduces mortality from 30% to 2–8%.

▸ **What does the clinician want to know?**
Severity of pulmonary artery involvement ● Origin of the thromboembolism ● Age of the thrombi.

Differential Diagnosis

Loss of volume, pneumonia	– Peripheral wedge-shaped density
	– Central vessel not detectable

Tips and Pitfalls

In loss of volume and pneumonia, differential diagnosis must include pulmonary embolism as it can be difficult to detect on CT scans where it occurs simultaneously with these entities.

Selected References

Interdisziplinäre S2-Leitlinie: Venenthrombose und Lungenembolie. VASA 2005; 34 (S66): 5–24

Mathis G et al. Thoracic ultrasound for diagnosing pulmonary embolism: a prospective multicenter study of 352 patients. Chest 2005; 128: 1531–1538

Schoepf UJ, Costello P. CT angiography for diagnosis of pulmonary embolism: state of the art. Radiology 2004; 230: 329–337

Stein PD et al. Multidetector computed tomography for acute pulmonary embolism. N Engl J Med 2006; 354: 2317–2327

Definition

▶ **Synonym**
Osler–Weber–Rendu disease.

▶ **Epidemiology**
Prevalence is 1 : 5000–8000 ● Varies widely according to geographic region ● No sex predilection.

▶ **Etiology, pathophysiology, pathogenesis**
Autosomal dominant disease of vascular connective tissue.
Two types of the disease are differentiated:
  – Endoglin gene on chromosome 9 (HHT-1) ● Pulmonary AVM occurs in 30–41 % of cases.
  – Activin receptorlike kinase-1 gene on chromosome 12 (HHT-2) ● Pulmonary AVM occurs in up to 14 % of cases.
  – Both forms lead to telangiectasia and AVMs of the skin and mucous membranes ● May also involve other organs (brain in 5–22 %, liver in 8–31 %, and gastrointestinal tract in 15–44 % of cases).

Imaging Signs

▶ **Modality of choice**
MRI for cerebral AVMs ● CT for AVMs outside the brain (especially lung and liver) ● The definitive modality is catheter angiography, which is also indispensable for planning treatment.

▶ **Standard chest radiograph findings**
Solitary or, less often, multiple well-demarcated round pulmonary focal lesions ● Broad vascular connections (bandlike densities) between the foci and the hilum.

▶ **Contrast echocardiography findings**
Screening modality for demonstrating pulmonary AVMs ● In a right-to-left shunt, studies performed after injection of an ultrasound contrast agent that does not pass into the lung immediately show contrast leakage into the left atrium and later into the left ventricle.

▶ **Color Doppler ultrasound findings**
Where there is liver involvement, even the B scan will show the increase in caliber of the feeders and draining vessels ● Flow volume in the celiac trunk and hepatic artery will often be increased ● Abnormal arteriovenous shunts will occasionally be directly visualized.

▶ **CT findings**
Pulmonary AVMs are visualized as round or tubular structures isodense to blood and with vascular connections to hilar vessels ● Abnormal vessels in the liver are readily detected.

▶ **MRI findings**
Abnormal feeders and draining veins in the central nervous system are visualized on noncontrast T1-weighted and T2-weighted sequences as tubular flow voids ● Contrast T1-weighted sequences show subcortical or subpial vascular changes as hyperintense linear or punctiform structures.

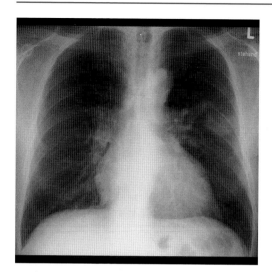

Fig. 4.27 Hereditary hemorrhagic telangiectasia. Standard chest radiograph. Barely visible lobulated shadow in the left midfield, connected to the hilum by a bandlike shadow.

▶ **CTA, MRA, and DSA findings**
Distinctive features of the vascular architecture of extracerebral AVMs are well visualized on CTA and MRA ● DSA provides the most precise imaging ● Because it is an invasive modality, DSA is usually used only for embolization.

Clinical Aspects

▶ **Typical presentation**
Epistaxis occurs in over 90% of all patients (usually the initial manifestation) ● Symptoms vary depending on the organs that are affected ● Dyspnea ● Cyanosis ● Cardiac failure ● Headache ● Seizures.

▶ **Therapeutic options**
Catheter embolization is the treatment of choice for visceral AVMs ● Additional surgical measures may be indicated.

▶ **Course and prognosis**
Visceral AVMs determine the clinical course ● Ischemic insults ● Cerebral abscesses ● Intracranial hemorrhages ● Heart failure ● Portosystemic encephalopathy ● Bleeding from varices ● Left untreated, symptomatic pulmonary AVMs are fatal in 4–22% of all cases and in up to 40% of severe cases ● The complication rate of pulmonary AVMs is increased during pregnancy.

▶ **What does the clinician want to know?**
Size of the visceral AVM ● Is embolization indicated?

Fig. 4.28 a, b CT after contrast administration (same patient as in **Fig. 4.27**). The transverse image shows round and tubular densities in the apical segment of left lower lobe (**a**). The coronal MIP reconstruction shows an extensive AVM fed by a dilated branch of the left pulmonary artery (**b**).

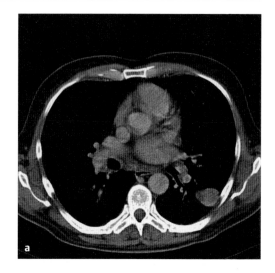

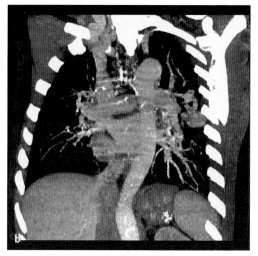

Differential Diagnosis

The diagnosis is made on the basis of the Curaçao criteria (epistaxis, telangiectasia, visceral lesions, and family history) • 70% of patients with pulmonary AVMs have underlying hereditary hemorrhagic telangiectasia • Only a small percentage of cerebral AVMs is associated with hereditary hemorrhagic telangiectasia.

Tips and Pitfalls

It is particularly important to exclude a pulmonary AVM prior to pregnancy.

Selected References

Buscarini E et al. Hepatic vascular malformations in hereditary hemorrhagic telangiectasia: imaging findings. AJR Am J Roentgenol 1994; 163: 1105–1110

Fulbright RK et al. MR of hereditary hemorrhagic telangiectasia: prevalence and spectrum of cerebrovascular malformations. AJNR Am J Neuroradiol 1998; 19: 477–484

Jaskolka J et al. Imaging of hereditary hemorrhagic telangiectasia. AJR Am J Roentgenol 2004; 307–314

Saluja S et al. Embolotherapy in the bronchial and pulmonary circulations. Radiol Clin North Am 2000; 38: 425–448

Definition

▶ **Epidemiology**
Occurs in 0.2–3% of the population.
▶ **Etiology, pathophysiology, pathogenesis**
Persistence of the postrenal segment of the left supracardinal vein ● This leads to development of two venous trunks inferior to the renal veins ● The left trunk drains into the left renal vein.

Imaging Signs

▶ **Modality of choice**
Incidental finding.

Clinical Aspects

▶ **Typical presentation**
Asymptomatic.
▶ **Therapeutic options**
None.
▶ **Course and prognosis**
No increased tendency to develop deep venous thrombosis in the pelvis or lower extremity.
▶ **What does the clinician want to know?**
Clinical significance for placement of an inferior vena cava filter, and surgical procedures in the retroperitoneal space.

Fig. 5.1 Illustration of double inferior vena cava.

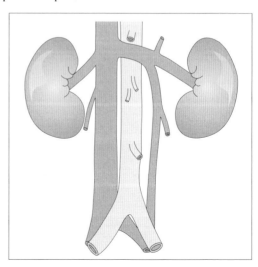

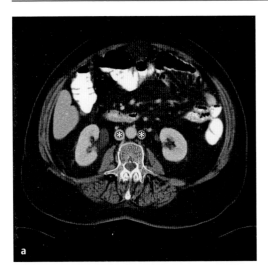

Fig. 5.2 a, b Contrast CT, axial (**a**) and coronal (**b**). Broad veins course on either side of the abdominal aorta (asterisks), linked by the left renal vein.

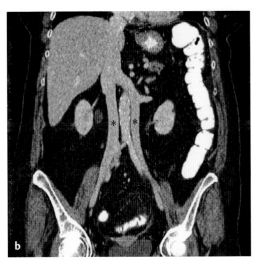

Differential Diagnosis

Retroperitoneal
lymphadenopathy

– CT shows slightly enhancing masses isodense to soft tissue

Tips and Pitfalls

Can be mistaken for a dilated left testicular or ovarian vein or enlarged retroperitoneal lymph nodes.

Selected References

Bass JE et al. Spectrum of congenital anomalies of the inferior vena cava: cross-sectional imaging findings. RadioGraphics 2000; 20: 639–652

Minniti S et al. Congenital anomalies of the venae cavae: embryological origin, imaging features and report of three new variants. Eur Radiol 2002; 12: 2040–2055

Definition

Localized increase in the aortic lumen by more than 50% • True aneurysm • Dilation involves all three layers of the aortic wall.

▶ **Epidemiology**

Typical finding in men aged 60–70 years • Prevalence in males is 1.3–8.9%, in females 1.0–2.2% • The three most important risk factors are age, sex, and smoking • Increased familial incidence suggests a genetic component • Often associated with iliac arterial aneurysms.

▶ **Etiology, pathophysiology, pathogenesis**

Biomechanical forces • Inflammation with increased formation of reactive oxygen radicals • Matrix enzymes react with metalloproteins, leading to proteolysis in the connective tissue.

Imaging Signs

▶ **Modality of choice**

Multidetector CT.

▶ **General findings**

Circumscribed or generalized dilation of the aorta • Focal dilation suggests mycotic or traumatic etiology • Lesion exhibits perfused and thrombotic components.

▶ **Ultrasound, color Doppler ultrasound findings**

Good modality for determining the size and evaluating the course of the lesion • Screening.

▶ **CTA and MRA findings**

Size is determined on MPRs • Relationship to the branches of the aorta is visualized • Crescentic calcification on CT • Inflammatory reaction in the surrounding fatty tissue • Modalities are useful for planning treatment • Blurring of the aortic wall • Signs of imminent perforation include increased density and extraluminal contrast medium in the thrombus or perivascular contrast medium.

▶ **DSA**

Only indicated where CTA or MRA of sufficient quality is unavailable or possibly in stent placement with a graduated catheter • Only visualizes the perfused component of the vessel • Failure to visualize the lumbar arteries is an indirect sign of a thrombus.

Table 5.1 Diagnostic values

Abdominal aorta	Outer diameter
Normal	1.8–2 cm
Aneurysm	> 3 cm

Fig. 5.3 Abdominal aortic aneurysm. CTA of the abdominal aorta. The maximum intensity projection (MIP) creates an image resembling DSA. The study demonstrates the extent of the infrarenal abdominal aortic aneurysm and involvement of the pelvic arteries.

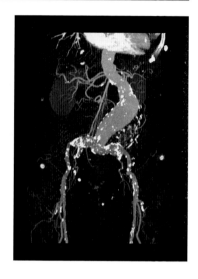

Clinical Aspects

▶ **Typical presentation**
Often asymptomatic • Abdominal pain • Back pain • Pulsations • Bimanual palpation detects 80% of abdominal aortic aneurysms over 5 cm in diameter.

▶ **Therapeutic options**
Elective treatment is indicated for lesions over 5 cm in diameter or which increase in size by more than 0.5 cm in 5 months • Open surgery with placement of a vascular prosthesis or stent placement.

▶ **Course and prognosis**
In its natural course, the disorder long remains asymptomatic until sudden and fatal rupture occurs • The rate of rupture depends on the diameter:
  – Below 5 cm, the risk is less than 1%
  – Above 5 cm, the risk is about 10%
  – Above 7 cm, the risk is over 30%
  – Thirty-day mortality for elective surgery is less than 6% • 5-year survival rate is 70%, with a high rate of comorbidity • 30-day mortality for stent graft is less than surgery and long-term survival is nearly identical to surgery.

▶ **What does the clinician want to know?**
Size of the abdominal aortic aneurysm for planning surgery or stent placement • Involvement of arterial origins • Evaluation of blood flow beyond the aneurysm • Dissection • Signs of imminent rupture.

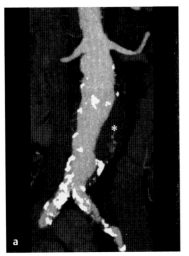 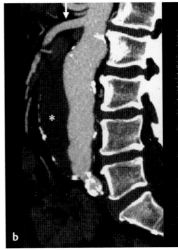

Fig. 5.4 a, b CTA of the abdominal aorta, coronal (**a**) and sagittal (**b**) reconstructions (MPR). The perfused and thrombosed components (asterisk) of the abdominal aortic aneurysm are clearly differentiated. The relationship to the renal arteries and superior mesenteric artery is also clearly visualized (arrow).

Differential Diagnosis

Dissecting aneurysm	– Turbulent hemorrhage in the aortic wall from an intimal tear – Aneurysmal dilation is not invariably present – Often begins in the chest
Penetrating ulcer	– Focal area of blood flow beneath atherosclerotic plaques and/or ulcer – Usually in the chest – Can lead to dissecting aneurysm
False aneurysm	– Surrounded only by adventitia and connective tissue – Usually a sequela of injury to the aortic wall
Mycotic abdominal aortic aneurysm	– Fever (50% of all cases), leukocytosis (80%), positive blood cultures – Rapidly increases in size – Lobulated saccular aneurysm – Pocket of air in the aortic wall – Periaortic abscess
Inflammatory abdominal aortic aneurysm	– See relevant section

Abdomen

Tips and Pitfalls

Incomplete visualization of the thoracic aorta, pelvic arteries, and drainage • Failure to exclude further aneurysms.

Selected References

Dock W et al. [Prevalence of abdominal aortic aneurysms: a sonographic screening study.] Rofo 1998; 168: 356–360 [In German]

Sakalihasan N et al. Abdominal aortic aneurysm. Lancet 2005; 365: 1577–1589

Singh K et al. Prevalence of and risk factors for abdominal aortic aneurysms. The Tromsø study. Am J Epidemiol 2001; 154: 236–244

Definition

▶ **Epidemiology**
Account for 5–15% of all abdominal aortic aneurysms ● Annual incidence rate is 0.1 : 100 000 ● Prevalence is 1.4 : 100 000 ● Commonly occurs in men between the ages of 50 and 60 years ● More than 80% of patients are smokers ● Males are affected 6–30 times more often than females.

▶ **Etiology, pathophysiology, pathogenesis**
Chronic periaortitis ● Inflammatory abdominal aortic aneurysm of variable severity ● Idiopathic retroperitoneal fibrosis (Ormond disease) ● Combination of both ● Chronic, nonspecific inflammation arising from the adventitia, containing lymphocytes and plasma cells, possibly a localized immune response to antigens from atherosclerotic plaques ● Thoracic aorta is involved in 10% of all cases ● Infrarenal aorta in 90% ● In 40%, pelvic arteries are also involved.

Imaging Signs

▶ **Modality of choice**
CT.

▶ **Ultrasound, color Doppler ultrasound findings**
Differentiates between aneurysmal lumen, thrombus, crescentic calcification, and surrounding retroperitoneal halo, which is usually hypoechoic ● Hydronephrosis.

▶ **CT findings**
Periaortic, primarily anterolateral soft tissue halo ● Aorta is not displaced anteriorly ● Fluid retention in periaortic fatty tissue ● Ureters may be encased ● Isodense to muscle on unenhanced scans ● Shows marked enhancement in the acute phase of inflammation ● Enhances less in the inactive phase ● Ureters are well visualized.

▶ **MRI findings**
– T1-weighted sequences show a hypointense periaortic soft tissue halo ● The inflammatory mass is sharply demarcated from the surrounding fatty tissue.
– T2-weighted sequences show hyperintense findings in the acute phase of inflammation ● Generally hypointense in the inactive stage.
– Normal caliber of the abdominal aorta is 1.8–2 cm ● Thickness of the periaortic halo is 0.5–3 cm.

Clinical Aspects

▶ **Typical presentation**
Fifty to 80% of cases present with abdominal and/or back pain ● Fever and weight loss occur in 20–50% ● Urinary stasis occurs in 10%, usually on the left side initially ● Extensive retroperitoneal fibrosis can lead to symptoms from compression of adjacent organs ● Laboratory findings include signs of acute inflammation.

Fig. 5.5 a, b Inflammatory abdominal aortic aneurysm. CT of the abdominal aorta (delayed image) (**a**). Anterolateral soft tissue halo (arrowheads), which also surrounds the left ureter and only enhances slightly. Left kidney with nephrostomy. CT (arterial phase) after 1 year (**b**). Slight enlargement of the periaortic soft tissue halo. Both ureters are splinted with double J catheters.

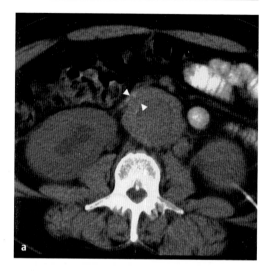

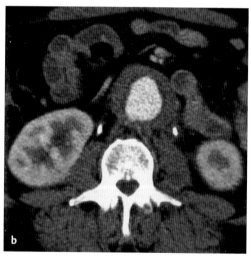

▶ **Therapeutic options**

Conservative therapy has high rates of failure and recurrence ● Open surgery with a vascular prosthesis ● Therapy of urinary stasis with ureter stent ● Stent placement may be considered (only individual case reports are available at present).

▶ **Course and prognosis**

Postoperative 30-day mortality is somewhat higher than in a normal abdominal aortic aneurysm ● Complete postoperative remission of the inflammatory tissue reaction is achieved in up to 55% of all cases ● The time frame for remission is months to years ● Lesion may recur ● Suture aneurysm occurs in up to 10% of all cases ● Therefore, follow-up examinations with CT or MRI are indicated.

▶ **What does the clinician want to know?**

Size of the aneurysm and inflammation (for planning surgery and stent placement) ● Involvement of arterial origins.

Differential Diagnosis

Nonidiopathic retroperitoneal fibrosis	– Causes include medication, drug use, radiation therapy, surgery, trauma, tumors (lymphoma, sarcoma), infections
	– Aneurysmal dilation is not invariably present
	– Aorta is often anteriorly displaced
Mycotic aneurysm	– Fever (50% of all cases), leukocytosis (80%), positive blood cultures
	– Rapidly increases in size
	– Lobulated saccular aneurysm
	– Pocket of air in the aortic wall
	– Periaortic abscess
Contained rupture	– Extraluminal contrast medium
	– No inflammatory fluid retention in periaortic fatty tissue
	– Periaortic soft tissue halo does not enhance
Takayasu arteritis	– Usually affects young women
	– Usually involves the thoracic aorta

Tips and Pitfalls

Failure to obtain delayed images can lead to insufficient demonstration of the ureters.

Selected References

Meier P et al. Rethinking the triggering inflammatory processes of chronic periaortitis. Nephron Exp Nephrol 2007; 105: e17–e23

Schmitz F et al. [Inflammatory aortic aneurysm after vascular-prosthetic treatment. Morphological findings after years of incorporation.] Pathologe 2004; 25: 120–126 [In German]

Tang T et al. Inflammatory abdominal aortic aneurysms. Eur J Vasc Endovasc Surg 2005; 29: 353–362

Vaglio A et al. Chronic periaortitis: a spectrum of diseases. Curr Opin Rheumatol 2005, 17: 34–40

Definition

▶ **Epidemiology**
Tenth most common cause of death in men over 55 years • Mortality is 60–80% • The high mortality has remained essentially unchanged for the past 20 years.

▶ **Etiology, pathophysiology, pathogenesis**
The risk of rupture depends on the diameter of the aneurysm • *Rupture rate for aneurysms:* < 5 cm, below 1%; > 5 cm, 10%; > 7 cm, over 30% • Risk factors include hypertension, chronic lung infection, gender, and smoking • 70% of ruptures are retroperitoneal, 25% occur in the abdominal cavity.

Imaging Signs

▶ **Modality of choice**
Multidetector CT.

▶ **Ultrasound, color Doppler ultrasound findings**
Unstable patient with abdominal aortic aneurysm and retroperitoneal hematoma • The site of the rupture itself cannot be directly visualized.

▶ **Multidetector CT findings**
Increasing size of the aneurysm is a sign of imminent rupture • Increased size of lumen relative to thrombus • Crescent of calcification is interrupted • Acute extravasation of contrast medium occurs in a rupture • Discontinuity of the aortic wall • Anterior displacement of the kidneys • Retroperitoneal hematoma • Hemorrhage spreads to other compartments • Aorta is masked by adjacent structures, usually along the posterior wall (sign of a contained rupture) • "Crescent sign" on unehanced CT scans—a hyperdense crescent in the thrombus consistent with acute hemorrhage • Contrast crescent within the thrombus on CTA.

Clinical Aspects

▶ **Typical presentation**
Sudden life-threatening emergency • 30–50% of patients die before reaching the hospital • Hypovolemic shock • Pulsating mid-abdominal mass • Less than 50% of patients exhibit the classic triad of symptoms—back pain, hypotension, and pulsation.

▶ **Therapeutic options**
Surgery involving reconstruction of the aorta with a vascular prosthesis; high 30-day mortality, on average 50% • Stent placement is increasingly used; 30-day mortality is around 20%.

▶ **Course and prognosis**
Mortality before reaching the hospital is 65% • 50% of patients reaching the hospital die • Those surviving 3 months post surgery have good prognosis.

▶ **What does the clinician want to know?**
Quick imaging and diagnosis are essential • Location of the rupture • Extent • Size • Involvement of aortic arterial branches.

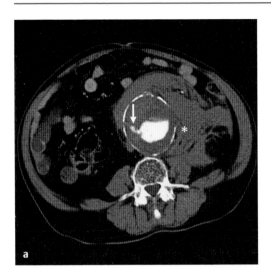

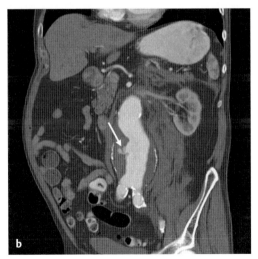

Fig. 5.6 a, b Rupture of an abdominal aortic aneurysm. CTA of the abdominal aorta, axial (**a**) and coronal (**b**) MPRs. Free fluid in the abdomen (asterisk) and contrast accumulation (arrow) in the thrombus communicating with the true lumen.

Differential Diagnosis

Acute abdomen	– Numerous causes
	– Many diagnoses can be excluded by CT
Mycotic aneurysm	– Lobulated contours
	– Saccular
	– Inflammatory halo, abscess around the aorta
	– Gas formation
	– Vertebral changes
Aortoenteric fistula	– Acute gastrointestinal hemorrhage, often preceded by a "warning hemorrhage"
	– Melena
	– Intraluminal or periaortic gas
Aortocaval fistula	– Heart failure and signs of a left-to-right shunt
	– Machine noise
	– Leg edema

Tips and Pitfalls

Delay in performing diagnostic procedures.

Selected References

Dore R et al. [Unusual CT features in ruptures of abdominal aortic aneurysms.] Rofo 1988; 148: 127–130 [In German]

Mehta M et al. Establishing a protocol for endovascular treatment of ruptured abdominal aortic aneurysms: outcomes of a prospective analysis. J Vasc Surg 2006; 44: 1–8

Rakita D et al. Spectrum of CT findings in rupture and impending rupture of abdominal aortic aneurysms. RadioGraphics 2007; 27: 497–507

Schwartz SA et al. CT findings of rupture, impending rupture, and contained rupture of abdominal aortic aneurysms. AJR Am J Roentgenol 2007; 188: W57–62

Definition

▶ **Epidemiology**
Endoleaks occur in 15–25% of cases ● Rupture rate of an ordinary abdominal aortic aneurysm after stent placement is less than 2%.

▶ **Etiology, pathophysiology, pathogenesis**
Endoleak: Persistent blood flow outside the stent and within the aneurysmal sac ● Incomplete decompression of the aneurysm ● Pulsatile pressure load ● No reduction of volume within the aneurysmal sac.

Imaging Signs

▶ **Modality of choice**
CT.

▶ **General findings**
Endovascular therapy of abdominal aortic aneurysm is an accepted alternative to surgery ● The objectives of regular follow-up examinations after stent placement include:
– Monitoring the size of the aneurysm
– Detecting and describing endoleaks
– Detecting mechanical changes in the stent graft (migration, kinking, fracture).
– The location of the contrast accumulation within the aneurysmal sac can suggest the type of endoleak:
– *Type 1:* At the proximal or distal end
– *Type 2:* Peripheral without contact with the stent ● Tubelike configuration adjacent to the aortic wall
– *Type 3:* Posteriorly from the lumbar arteries ● Halo around the stent

▶ **Ultrasound findings**
Not suitable for routine follow-up after stent placement ● Contrast ultrasound may be used to detect slow-flowing endoleaks (type 2) and for correct classification.

▶ **CT findings**
Arterial phase visualizes the arteries supplying the endoleak and early extravasation of contrast agent ● The late phase (60 seconds after the arterial phase) shows contrast accumulation in the aneurysmal sac ● MPRs can be used to measure size over time.

▶ **MRA**
May only be used where the stent material does not produce artifacts ● Quality is at least equivalent to DSA ● Time-of-flight MRA techniques and intravascular contrast may be helpful.

▶ **DSA**
Rarely necessary to detect endoleaks, but useful for correctly classifying them (error rate of CTA is 14%) ● Technique involves aortography with the catheter advanced proximally and distally into the main body of the stent, and into the superior mesenteric arteries and both iliac arteries where indicated.

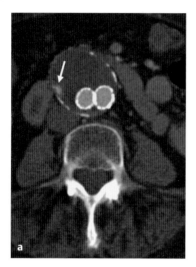
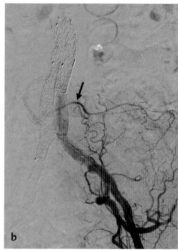

Fig. 5.7a, b Endoleak type 2. CT, arterial phase (**a**). Contrast accumulation (arrow) in the periphery of an abdominal aortic aneurysm after stent placement. DSA, catheter in the left branch of the graft (**b**). Endoleak is filled via a lumbar artery (arrow).

Clinical Aspects

▶ **Typical presentation**
Asymptomatic • Objective of regular follow-up examinations is to detect imminent rupture.

▶ **Therapeutic options**
– *Type 1:* Immediate treatment • Angioplasty • Stent or extension of the stent graft.
– *Type 2:* Indication is controversial • Treatment is indicated only where the aneurysmal sac increases in size • Embolization.
– *Type 3:* Immediate treatment • Placement of an additional stent to stop the leak.
– *Type 4:* Rare • No treatment.
– *Type 5:* Intensive search for endoleak • Where the search is negative and the aneurysm increases in size, open surgery is indicated.

▶ **Course and prognosis**
Thirty-day mortality after elective stent placement is 1.7–3.5% • 2-year mortality is about 15% • Type 1 and 3 endoleaks require immediate treatment • Type 2 has a high rate of spontaneous occlusion.

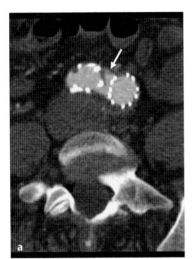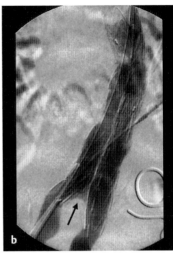

Fig. 5.8 a, b Endoleak type 1. CT, arterial phase (**a**). Contrast accumulation (arrow) in the distal part of an abdominal aortic aneurysm after stent placement. The right iliac branch is too short. DSA, catheter in the main body of the stent graft (**b**). Distal filling of the endoleak (arrow).

▶ **What does the clinician want to know?**

Size of the aneurysm over time ● Mechanical changes in the stent graft ● Diagnosis and classification of an endoleak.

Differential Diagnosis

Endoleak type 1	– Leak at the anchoring point of the stent graft
Endoleak type 2	– Leak through collateral arteries
Endoleak type 3	– Leak through stent graft defect
Endoleak type 4	– Porosity of the stent graft
Endoleak type 5	– Internal tension

Tips and Pitfalls

Failure to obtain images in the late phase.

Selected References

Pitton MB et al. [Classification and treatment of endoleaks after endovascular treatment of abdominal aortic aneurysms.] Fortschr Röntgenstr 2005; 177: 24–34 [In German]

Seifarth H, Kraemer S. [Endovascular therapy for ruptured aneurysms: Pre- and postinterventional diagnostic imaging.] Rofo 2008; 180: 223–230 [In German]

Stavropoulos SW, Charagundla SR. Imaging techniques for detection and management of endoleaks after endovascular aortic aneurysm repair. Radiology 2007; 243: 641–655

Stolzmann P et al. Endoleaks after endovascular abdominal aortic aneurysm repair: detection with dual-energy dual-source CT. Radiology 2008; 249: 682–691

Definition

▶ **Epidemiology**
Atherosclerotic occlusions and stenoses are usually present • Isolated involvement of the aorta is common; usually occurring in combination with iliac involvement • In Germany, peripheral arterial occlusive disease affects 2.2% of men and 1.8% of women.

▶ **Etiology, pathophysiology, pathogenesis**
The main causes are the primary risk factors of atherosclerosis • Smoking • Diabetes • Disorders of fat metabolism • Hypertension • Age.
Small aorta syndrome is a particularly malignant special case in younger female smokers younger than 55, often associated with significant nicotine misuse.

Imaging Signs

▶ **Modality of choice**
Multidetector CT • MRI.

▶ **General findings**
Focal stenosis or occlusion of the abdominal aorta • Often posterior and close to the bifurcation • Usually large collaterals • Significant calcifications • In small aorta syndrome, findings often include a slender aorta and pelvic arteries and a high bifurcation.

▶ **Color Doppler ultrasound findings**
Accelerated blood flow in the stenosis • Poststenotic turbulence and limited spectral window • Ultrasound in the pelvis is often limited by bowel gas and obesity • Visualizing complex vascular courses is difficult and time-consuming.

▶ **CTA and MRA findings**
Stenoses and collaterals are usually well visualized • Vascular calcification can be readily evaluated on CTA • Calcifications in the central vessels are less of a problem than peripheral calcifications as the vascular lumens are usually large in relation to the calcification plaques • This produces fewer artifacts on the primary images and simplifies image processing with slices selected according to the course of the vessel.

▶ **DSA findings**
Indicated where CTA or MRA of sufficient quality is unavailable and where immediate percutaneous treatment is being considered • Arterial DSA in aortic occlusion is limited to transaxillary or transbrachial approaches • In a small aorta, lumen diameter will be < 1.2 cm (normal value is 1.8–2 cm).

Clinical Aspects

▶ **Typical presentation**
Intermittent claudication • Ischemic pain at rest is rare as collateral circulation is usually adequate • Small aorta syndrome is characterized by the triad of a young female smoker, involvement of the distal abdominal aorta, and presence of severe calcifications.

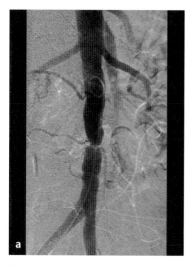
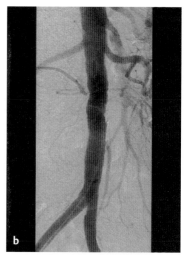

Fig. 5.9 a, b Chronic occlusive disease of the aorta. DSA. High-grade stenosis of the abdominal aorta at the level of vertebra L3. Before (**a**) and after (**b**) percutaneous balloon angioplasty and stent placement.

Fig. 5.10 A 48-year-old female smoker with occlusion of the abdominal aorta close to the bifurcation and well developed collaterals. DSA. The caliber of the infrarenal aorta and pelvic arteries is too small.

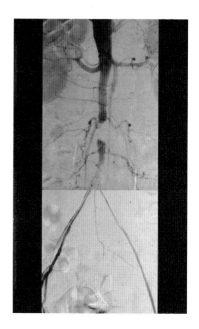

▶ **Therapeutic options**
Risk factors should be reduced and conservative treatment attempted ● Intolerable claudication is treated with angioplasty and, in applicable cases, stent placement ● Open surgical revascularization (endarterectomy, aortobifemoral bypass) should be considered in addition to angioplasty, especially where the aortoiliac vessels have small lumens.

Differential Diagnosis

Leriche syndrome	– Often affects male smokers aged 30–40 years
Takayasu arteritis	– Often affects women under 40 years
	– Hypertension
	– Focal involvement with aneurysm
	– Also affects other medium and large arteries
	– Generalized symptoms (acute) and neurologic symptoms (late)
Atypical coarctation	– Males under 20 years
	– Presumably congenital

Selected References

Caes F et al. Small artery syndrome in women. Surg Gynecol Obstet 1985; 161: 165–170

Poncyljusz W et al. Primary stenting in the treatment of focal atherosclerotic abdominal aortic stenoses. Clin Radiol 2006; 61: 691–695

Walton BL et al. Percutaneous intervention for the treatment of hypoplastic aortoiliac syndrome. Catheter Cardiovasc Interv 2003; 60: 329–334

Definition
. . . .

Synonym: Complete obliteration of the aortic bifurcation.

► **Epidemiology**
Rare special case of peripheral arterial occlusive disease.

► **Etiology, pathophysiology, pathogenesis**
Occurs in the setting of peripheral arterial occlusive disease ● Occlusion of the infrarenal aorta including the bifurcation ● Initially involves aortic stenosis ● Later progresses to occlusion from additional thromboses ● Peripheral perfusion is usually maintained by well-developed collaterals in the chest and abdominal wall.

Imaging Signs
. . . .

► **Modality of choice**
CTA ● MRA.

► **Pathognomonic findings**
Occlusion of the infrarenal aorta, including the bifurcation and common iliac arteries ● Distal filling occurs through well-developed collaterals in the chest and abdominal wall.

► **Color Doppler ultrasound findings**
Aortic occlusion is usually well visualized ● Limited visualization of the collaterals.

► **CTA and MRA findings**
The collaterals and distal blood flow are very clearly visualized due to the intravenous contrast filling of all arteries.

► **DSA findings**
Axillary approach is necessary ● The collaterals and distal blood flow are usually visualized incompletely, depending on the position of the catheter.

Clinical Aspects
. . . .

► **Typical presentation**
Bilateral symptoms of peripheral arterial occlusive disease (stages II–IV) ● Impotence ● Bilateral acute ischemia syndrome may occur.

► **Therapeutic options**
Aortobifemoral bypass ● Percutaneous transluminal angioplasty with stent.

► **Course and prognosis**
After surgical treatment, 85% of patients survive 5 years and 55% survive 10 years.

► **What does the clinician want to know?**
Extent of the occlusion ● Degree of collateralization ● Other stenoses or occlusive lesions of the leg arteries ● Renal arterial stenosis.

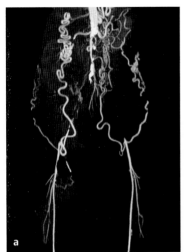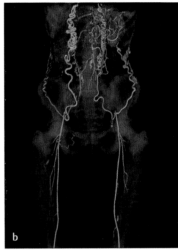

Fig. 5.11 a, b Leriche syndrome. CTA. Occlusion of the infrarenal aorta including the bifurcation and both common iliac arteries. Filling of the external iliac arteries occurs through well-developed collaterals in the abdominal wall.

Differential Diagnosis

High-grade stenosis of the aorta and/or bifurcation — Partially patent lumen with perfusion

Tips and Pitfalls

The acquisition plane on CTA can overtake the contrast bolus in the legs where arterial flow is slow due to occlusion • This problem may be minimized by reducing the speed of table movement • With DSA a catheter position in the ascending aorta can improve visualization of runoff vessels.

Selected References

Carrafiello G et al. Endovascular treatment of steno-occlusions of the infrarenal abdominal aorta. Radiol Med 2006; 111: 949–958

Mavioglu I et al. Surgical management of chronic total occlusion of abdominal aorta. J Cardiovasc Surg (Torino) 2003; 44: 87–93

Ruehm SG et al. Contrast-enhanced MR angiography in patients with aortic occlusion (Leriche syndrome). J Magn Reson Imaging 2000; 11: 401–410

Definition

▶ **Epidemiology**
Usually occurs in patients over age 60 suffering from multiple disorders • Accounts for 1 % of all patients admitted with acute abdominal pain • Accounts for 0.5 % of all emergency abdominal operations • Occurs in 2 % of all patients after aortic surgery • Nonocclusive form frequently occurs in heart surgery and in dialysis patients.

▶ **Etiology, pathophysiology, pathogenesis**
Acute reduction of blood circulation in the visceral arteries • Reduced blood circulation and vasospasms with intact circulation in larger vessels • Ischemia (local RR < 40 mmHg) lasting more than 15 minutes leads to structural changes and impaired microcirculation • Changes are initially reversible but then progress to transmural necrosis, peritonitis, and sepsis.

  – Occlusive mesenteric ischemia involves local thrombosis in 30 % of all cases, usually adjacent to the ostium • Embolism occurs in 25 %, of these: 15 % at the origin, 50 % in the first 3–10 cm, and 35 % distal; 80 % of all cases involve the superior mesenteric artery • Mesenteric vein thrombosis occurs in 15 %.
  – Nonocclusive mesenteric ischemia accounts for 25 % of all cases of mesenteric ischemia.
  – Other causes include bowel obstruction • Vasculitis • Compression • Trauma.

Imaging Signs

▶ **Modality of choice**
Multidetector CT.

▶ **Color Doppler ultrasound findings**
Absence of Doppler signals suggests visceral arterial occlusion • Ileus often renders examination impossible • The inferior mesenteric artery is not visualized • *Caution:* Time delay.

▶ **Multidetector CT findings**
This new gold standard visualizes the mesenteric vessels (CTA), bowel, and other abdominal organs • CT must be immediately available • Oral administration of water or methyl cellulose for bowel contrast is indicated wherever feasible.

  – Specific signs include direct visualization of the arterial occlusion and/or mesenteric vein thrombosis • The bowel wall does not enhance.
  – Nonspecific signs include bowel distension • Thickening of the bowel wall • Hyperperfusion • Delayed filling of a segment of the bowel • Persistent enhancement in the late phase • Pneumatosis • Free air • Ascites.

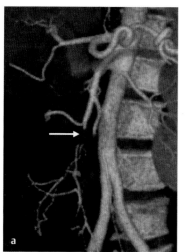

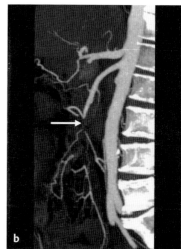

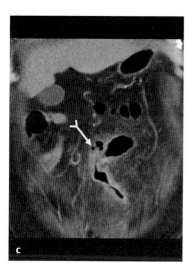

Fig. 5.12 a–c Acute mesenteric ischemia in occlusion of the superior mesenteric artery (arrow). Multidetector CT, arterial phase. Volume rendering (**a**) and MIP (**b**) images both show filling of the distal branches of the superior mesenteric artery via the right colic artery. The coronal MPR (**c**) shows hyperemia of a small bowel segment, mesenteric inflammation, and free air (forked arrow) consistent with perforation.

Fig. 5.13 Selective DSA of the superior mesenteric artery showing embolic occlusion of the ileocolic artery (arrow) and jejunal arteries (arrowhead). Filling of the distal ileocolic artery via collaterals from the proximal jejunal arteries and right colic artery.

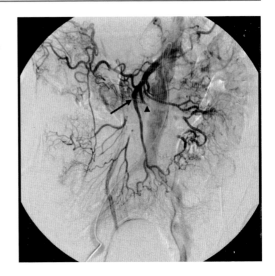

▶ **DSA findings**

Indicated where multidetector CT findings are nonspecific or equivocal ● Modality of choice for nonocclusive mesenteric ischemia, showing narrowing of the branches of the superior mesenteric artery ● Simultaneous dilation and stenosis produces a "string of pearls" pattern ● Vasospasms in the vascular arcades of the bowel ● Impaired filling of the intramural vessels ● Slow arterial flow (up to 20 seconds) ● Delayed filling of the mesenteric veins ● Intraarterial papaverine is a therapeutic option ● Thickness of the distended bowel wall is less than 3 mm.

Clinical Aspects

▶ **Typical presentation**

The typical patient is over 60 with abdominal pain and heart disease ● In acute embolism the proximal superior mesenteric artery typically exhibits a three-phase course with sudden onset, temporary improvement, and severe generalized symptoms ● Depending on collateralization, symptoms in thrombosis and peripheral embolism may range from nonspecific muscle tension and insidious abdominal pain to the full picture of acute abdomen ● 30% of all cases involve vomiting, diarrhea, and fever ● Nonocclusive mesenteric ischemia has a high rate of comorbidity.

▶ **Therapeutic options**

Resection of irreversibly damaged bowel • Embolectomy • Thrombectomy • By-pass • Endovascular therapy without laparotomy and inspection of the bowel is problematic (see case studies) • Papaverine infusion is indicated for nonocclusive mesenteric ischemia.

▶ **Course and prognosis**

Mortality in embolic occlusion is 70% • Mortality in more central thrombosis in the superior mesenteric artery is 80–90% • Mortality in nonocclusive mesenteric ischemia is 90% • Surgery within 24 hours reduces mortality by 20%.

▶ **What does the clinician want to know?**

Location of the occlusion • Cause of the occlusion • Complications.

Differential Diagnosis

Mesenteric vein thrombosis	– Severe thickening of the bowel wall up to 15 mm – Usually visualized on ultrasound and multi-detector CT
Local ischemia due to strangulation	– Multidetector CT with MPRs can usually identify the cause – Typical course of the affected vessel
Inflammatory bowel disease	– Normal vascular anatomy – Hyperemia – Mixed picture with thickening of the bowel wall and stenosis

Tips and Pitfalls

Delay in performing multidetector CT studies due to unnecessary waiting time or initiating time-consuming diagnostic studies.

Selected References

Horton KM, Fishman EK. Multidetector CT angiography in the diagnosis of mesenteric ischemia. Radiol Clin North Am 2007; 45: 275–288

Kirkpatrick ID et al. Biphasic CT with mesenteric CT angiography in the evaluation of acute mesenteric ischemia: Initial experience. Radiology 2003; 229: 91–98

Kraemer SC et al. [Nonocclusive mesenteric ischemia: Radiologic diagnosis and treatment.] Rofo 2003; 175: 1177–1183 [In German]

Levy AD. Mesenteric ischemia. Radiol Clin North Am 2007; 45: 593–599

Definition

▶ **Epidemiology**
Autopsy statistics show that well over 50% of people older than 50 years have stenosis of visceral arteries.

▶ **Etiology, pathophysiology, pathogenesis**
Atherosclerosis is the cause in 90% of cases • Less common causes include congenital conditions, vasculitis, fibromuscular dysplasia, external vascular compression, and trauma • Functional ischemia due to cardiovascular insufficiency and external compression of the celiac trunk • Chronic, slowly progressive stenoses are compensated for by an extensive network of collaterals.

Imaging Signs

▶ **Modality of choice**
Color Doppler ultrasound • CTA • MRA.

▶ **General findings**
Narrowing of the lumen or occlusion of the mesenteric artery • Poststenotic dilation • Often occurs at the origin of the artery on the abdominal aorta and at bifurcations • Collaterals • Occlusion of the celiac trunk produces retrograde flow in the common hepatic artery.

▶ **Color Doppler ultrasound findings**
Well suited for screening the superior mesenteric artery and celiac trunk • Low sensitivity, but high specificity for stenosis and occlusion • Over 75% stenosis is present where systolic peak velocity in the superior mesenteric artery in a fasting patient exceeds 280 cm/s, and exceeds 200 cm/s in the celiac trunk • Functional test involves color Doppler ultrasound before and 45 minutes after a standardized test meal • Perfusion normally increases by 30%, but this does not occur in chronic mesenteric arterial stenosis or occlusion • Dynamic examination identifies respiration-dependent changes in the celiac trunk.

▶ **CTA**
Technical requirements include multislice CT • Rapid intravenous contrast injection • Oral contrast is contraindicated • Often the main trunk and first- to third-order branches are visualized • Aortic calcifications can be readily evaluated.

▶ **MRA**
Technical requirements include rapid intravenous contrast injection and fast data acquisition • Functional test involves MRI with phase-contrast imaging before and 45 minutes after a standardized test meal • Examination is performed at inspiration and expiration to identify respiration-dependent changes in the celiac trunk.

▶ **DSA**
Minimally invasive • Indicated only where CTA or MRA of sufficient quality is unavailable, where branches with small lumens must be visualized, and where immediate percutaneous treatment is being considered • Examination is performed at inspiration and expiration to identify respiration-dependent changes.

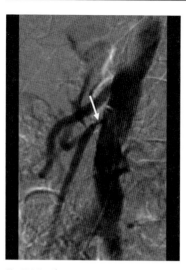

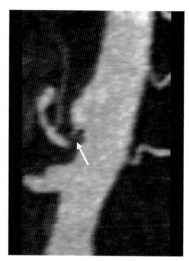

Fig. 5.14 Chronic mesenteric ischemia. DSA prior to angioplasty. High-grade stenosis of the superior mesenteric artery (arrow).

Fig. 5.15 Contrast MRA showing high-grade stenosis of the celiac trunk (arrow) close to the ostium.

Clinical Aspects

▶ **Typical presentation**

Often asymptomatic • Abdominal angina usually occurs only where two or three aortic branches are affected • Colicky abdominal pain occurs 15 minutes after eating • Weight loss due to malabsorption syndrome or disturbed motility • Epigastric flow sounds • Where there is collateral circulation via the internal iliac artery, exercising the legs can cause abdominal pain due to a steal effect.

▶ **Therapeutic options**

Elective treatment is indicated in symptomatic patients as emergency treatment of acute mesenteric ischemia has a mortality of 40–60% • Interventional treatment with angioplasty, with stent placement where indicated • Bypass • Endarterectomy.

▶ **Course and prognosis**

Natural course is progressive where atherosclerotic lesions are present • Symptoms recur in 20% of cases after treatment • Percutaneous transluminal angioplasty with stent has a slightly lower initial patency rate than surgery and requires repeated intervention earlier • Assisted patency rates are comparable for PTA and surgery.

▶ **What does the clinician want to know?**

Complications of ischemia ● Inflow is important to know prior to revascularization ● Extent of stenosis and occlusion ● Anastomosis sites for bypass surgery ● Drainage ● Portal venous system.

Differential Diagnosis
....

Compression syndrome (arcuate ligament of the diaphragm)	– Compression of the celiac trunk in expiration – Intermittent pain of uncertain causes – May be due to mechanical nerve irritation – Unrelated to eating
Acute mesenteric ischemia	– Acute onset of abdominal pain – Usually due to embolism of the superior mesenteric artery – Abrupt vascular occlusion, usually at bifurcations – Slight atherosclerotic changes in the vascular wall

Tips and Pitfalls
....

Examination of the celiac trunk in expiration is often neglected.

Selected References

Atkins MD et al. Surgical revascularization versus endovascular therapy for chronic mesenteric ischemia: a comparative experience. J Vasc Surg 2007; 45: 1162–1171

Cademartiri F et al. Multi-detector row CT angiography in patients with abdominal angina. RadioGraphics 2004; 24: 969–984

Otte JA et al. What is the best diagnostic approach for chronic gastrointestinal ischemia? Am J Gastroenterol 2007; 102: 2005–2010.

Definition

▶ **Epidemiology**
Heterogeneous group of disorders with varying regional incidence.

▶ **Etiology, pathophysiology, pathogenesis**
Unspecific inflammation of the vascular wall, often with necrosis and luminal narrowing ● Any vessel can be affected ● Immune complex vasculitides, pauci-immune or ANCA-associated vasculitides, and T-cell–mediated vasculitides ● The Chapel Hill system classifies disease according to the size of vessel primarily affected in combination with histologic findings or nosology (primary versus secondary forms; here vasculitis is considered part of a higher-order disease).

Imaging Signs

▶ **Modality of choice**
CT ● MRI ● DSA.

▶ **CT and MRI findings**
Dilated bowel loops ● Focal or diffuse thickening of the bowel wall ● Submucosal edema and hemorrhage ● Abnormal contrast enhancement of the bowel wall ● Stasis in mesenteric blood vessels ● Honeycomb configuration of blood vessels ("honeycomb sign") ● Ascites ● Lymphadenopathy ● Young patients exhibit signs of ischemia at unusual locations (stomach, duodenum, rectum), and in the small and large bowel simultaneously ● Irregular thickened arterial wall ● Vascular stenosis ● Poststenotic dilation ● Aneurysms ● Occlusion ● Increased collateralization ● Vascular findings may also be detectable on CTA and MRA, depending on their size and location.

▶ **DSA findings**
For additionally visualizing subtle findings in the mesenteric arterial microvasculature ● Small aneurysms ● Changes resembling a string of pearls ● Stenosis.

Clinical Aspects

▶ **Typical presentation**
Generalized symptoms include weight loss, weakness, myalgias, and fever ● Other symptoms specific to various vasculitides also occur ● Diagnosis is often made on the basis of a combination of clinical, histologic, and immune serology findings ● Typical complications include nonspecific paralytic ileus, mesenteric ischemia, perforations, and strictures.

▶ **Therapeutic options**
General measures ● Glucocorticoids ● Immunosuppressives.

▶ **What does the clinician want to know?**
Consider this disorder in patients with atypical findings ● Confirm the diagnosis where findings are unclear.

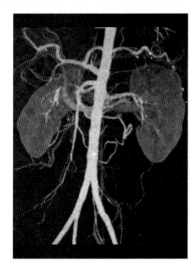

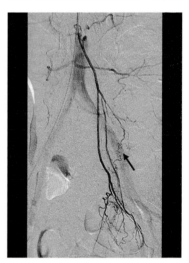

Fig. 5.16   Vasculitis involving the mesenteric arteries. CTA of the superior mesenteric artery. The artery resembles a string of pearls, exhibiting aneurysms and occlusions.

Fig. 5.17   DSA of the inferior mesenteric artery showing multiple occlusions and corkscrew arteries (arrow).

Differential Diagnosis

Large arteries: *Takayasu arteritis*	– Typical findings include involvement of the aortic arch in women younger than 50 years – Loss of pulse in the upper extremity – Involves the abdominal aorta and its branches in 32% of cases – Irregular thickened arterial wall, stenosis, aneurysms, occlusion
Medium arteries: *polyarteritis nodosa*	– Men aged 40–50 years – Multiple aneurysms up to 1 cm (present in 50% of all cases) are not pathognomonic as they also occur in other vasculitides – Kidney 85%, gastrointestinal tract 60%, liver 50%, spleen 45%, pancreas 30% – Small bowel is involved more often than mesentery and large bowel – Two-thirds of patients have gastrointestinal symptoms—bleeding (6%), perforation (5%), mesenteric infarction (1.4%)

Small arteries: Wegener granulomatosis	– Granulomatous respiratory tract inflammation – Necrotizing glomerulonephritis – Bowel involvement in 25 % of all cases, usually asymptomatic
Churg–Strauss syndrome	– Vasculitis of the respiratory tract – Extrapulmonary manifestations in the bowel, spleen, and heart, rarely in the kidney – Stomach, bowel—inflammation, ulcers, perforation, and bleeding
Microscopic polyangiitis	– Necrotizing glomerulonephritis (in 90 % of cases) and pulmonary involvement are common – Stomach, bowel—inflammation, ulcers, and bleeding
Henoch–Schönlein purpura	– Primarily affects boys under 10 years – Exanthema with maculopapules, fever, joint swelling – Stomach, bowel—edema and intramural hematoma, less often necrosis
Systemic lupus erythematosus	– Women aged 20–40 years – Autoimmune disorder – Stomach, bowel—inflammation with ischemia, bleeding, ileus, ulceration, infarction, and perforation affecting the entire gastrointestinal tract but primarily the area supplied by the superior mesenteric artery
Segmental arterial mediolysis (SAM)	– Noninflammatory, nonatherosclerotic vascular disease, most common in splanchnic arteries – Uncertain etiology, may be a form of fibromuscular dysplasia

Tips and Pitfalls

Arthritic, myalgic, intestinal, nervous, renal, cardiac, and pulmonary signs often lead to misdiagnosis.

Selected References

Gaubitz M, Domschke W. [Intestinal vasculitis—a diagnostic-therapeutic challenge.] Z Gastroenterol 2000; 38: 181–192 [In German]

Ha HK et al. Radiologic features of vasculitis involving the gastrointestinal tract. RadioGraphics 2000; 20: 779–794

Definition

▶ **Epidemiology**
Found in 0.07–10% of all autopsies • Splenic artery: 60% • Hepatic artery: 20% • Superior mesenteric artery: 6% • Celiac trunk: 4% • Gastric artery: 4% • Gastro-epiploic artery: 4% • Intestinal branches: 3% • Pancreaticoduodenal artery: 2% • Gastroduodenal artery: 1.5% • Inferior mesenteric artery: 0.5% • Multiple occurrences • Splenic artery aneurysms are the only aneurysms that occur more often in females than in males (ratio of 4 : 1) • In over 80% of cases, the affected patients are multiparous women.

▶ **Etiology, pathophysiology, pathogenesis**
Degeneration of the media • Hemodynamic factors • Vasculitides • Embolic-mycotic causes • Atherosclerosis is only a secondary cause • Aneurysms of the splenic artery occur more often with portal hypertension, after liver transplantation, and during pregnancy • False aneurysms after trauma or erosion of the arterial wall occur in pancreatitis or chronic ulcer.

Imaging Signs

▶ **Modality of choice**
CT.

▶ **Color Doppler ultrasound findings**
Hypoechoic round or fusiform area • Turbulent flow profile.

▶ **CT findings**
Focal dilation of the vascular lumen, which enhances markedly with contrast • Wall calcifications and partial thromboses commonly occur • Modality provides detailed information about vascular morphology and topography through the use of various projection techniques.

▶ **MRI**
Contrast 3D MRA provides diagnostic information of a quality comparable to CTA • The longer examination time is a disadvantage.

▶ **DSA**
No longer required for purely diagnostic purposes • Only indicated in combination with endovascular therapy.

Clinical Aspects

▶ **Typical presentation**
Often asymptomatic or showing only nonspecific symptoms • A rupture is the first clinical manifestation in 25% of all cases • Rupture into the abdominal cavity leads to acute abdomen • Penetration into the gastrointestinal tract, pancreatic duct, or a pancreatic pseudocyst may occur.

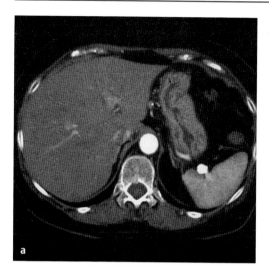

Fig. 5.18 a–d Aneurysm of the splenic artery. CT showing a partially calcified aneurysm in the splenic hilum in the arterial (**a**) and portal venous (**b**) contrast phases.

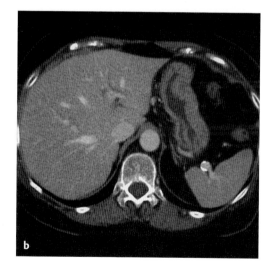

Fig. 5.18 c, d ▶

DSA (**c, d**). The same aneurysm before (**c**) and after coil embolization (**d**).

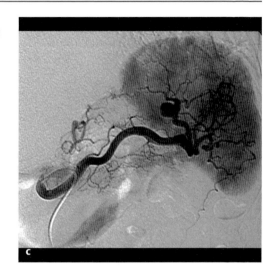

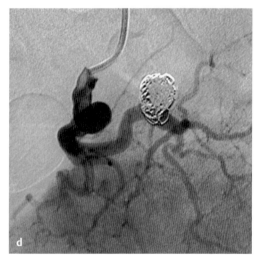

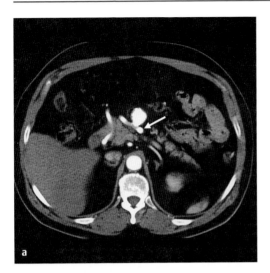

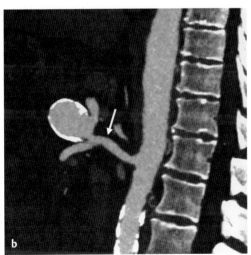

Fig. 5.19 a, b   Aneurysm of the superior mesenteric artery. CT. Axial source image (**a**) and sagittal MIP reconstruction (**b**). Crescentic calcified aneurysm at the bifurcation of the superior mesenteric artery (arrow) and a well developed collateral with simultaneous occlusion of the celiac trunk.

▶ **Therapeutic options**

Aneurysms exceeding 2 cm in diameter require treatment ● Follow-up examinations every 6 months are indicated for smaller aneurysms ● Endovascular or surgical treatment may be indicated depending on the location of the aneurysm and the patient's clinical condition.

▶ **Course and prognosis**

Incidence of rupture varies according to the location and underlying disorder ● Hepatic artery: 80% ● Superior mesenteric artery: 38–50% ● Celiac trunk: 13% ● Splenic artery: 3–10% ● Splenic artery aneurysms are particular prone to rupture during or after pregnancy (risk of rupture is 25–45%).

▶ **What does the clinician want to know?**

Localization ● Size ● Signs of imminent rupture.

Differential Diagnosis

Increased tortuosity of the splenic artery	– Best differentiated from an aneurysm on multiplanar CTA reconstructions, using volume-rendering technique where indicated
Islet cell tumor of the pancreas	– Highly vascularized tumor – Marked enhancement in the arterial phase – No vessel supplying or draining the lesion

Tips and Pitfalls

A splenic artery aneurysm can be misinterpreted as increased tortuosity of the splenic artery.

Selected References

Agrawal GA et al. Splenic artery aneurysms and pseudoaneurysms: clinical distinctions and CT appearances. AJR Am J Roentgenol 2007; 188: 992–999

Berceli SA. Hepatic and splenic artery aneurysms. Semin Vasc Surg 2005; 18: 196–201

Chiesa R et al. Visceral artery aneurysms. Ann Vasc Surg 2005; 19: 42–48

Croner RS et al. [Visceral artery anuerysms.] Dtsch Arztebl 2006; 103: A1367–1371 [In German]

Grego FG et al. Visceral artery aneurysms: a single center experience. Cardiovasc Surg 2003; 11: 19–25

Messina LM, Shanley CJ. Visceral artery aneurysms. Surg Clin North Am 1997; 77: 425–442

Definition

▶ **Epidemiology**

Incidence increases with age ● Risk is particularly high in people over 80 years ● Occurs in the upper gastrointestinal tract in 80% of cases and in the lower tract in 20%.

▶ **Etiology, pathophysiology, pathogenesis**

In upper gastrointestinal bleeding, the source of bleeding is proximal to the ligament of Treitz ● In lower gastrointestinal bleeding, the source is distal to the ligament of Treitz ● Most common causes include bleeding from esophageal varices ● Hemorrhagic gastritis ● Peptic ulcers ● Postoperative bleeding (especially after liver or pancreatic surgery ● Colonic diverticulum ● Angiodysplasia ● Tumors ● Ulcerative colitis ● Hemorrhoids ● Anal fissures ● Risk of bleeding is increased in patients on anticoagulants (warfarin, platelet aggregation inhibitors) ● Acute gastrointestinal bleeding with high blood flow affects circulation and can lead to hypovolemic shock ● Chronic gastrointestinal bleeding with low blood flow does not usually affect circulation but leads to anemia.

Imaging Signs

▶ **Modality of choice**

Endoscopy, although it may prove impossible to identify the source of massive bleeding ● Radiologic studies to identify the source of bleeding are indicated only when gastroscopy and colonoscopy are unsuccessful ● Radiologic modalities of choice are CTA, nuclear imaging, and DSA ● MRA using bloodpool agents is being evaluated.

▶ **Pathognomonic findings**

Contrast extravasation in the bowel lumen ● All imaging modalities can detect bleeding in only about 50% of cases as it may be below the detection threshold and intermittent bleeding may cease during the examination ● It is crucial to perform diagnostic imaging as quickly as possible after clinical onset of bleeding ● Where initial findings are negative, sensitivity can be increased by provocation with heparin or recombinant tissue plasminogen activator ● Probability of detection increases with an acute decrease in hemoglobin and hemodynamically significant bleeding ● Radiologic studies to identify the source of bleeding will usually be successful only in significant acute bleeding ● Radiologic modalities except nuclear imaging are not indicated as the initial study for chronic low-flow bleeding with melena.

▶ **CT findings**

The sensitivity of multidetector CT in detecting gastrointestinal bleeding is comparable with that of DSA ● Reconstructions from 3D CTA can usually demonstrate the arterial feeders ● The advantage over DSA is that it is a noninvasive modality readily available around the clock ● The technique involves a high intravenous dose, concentration, and injection rate of contrast agent (120–150 mL, 400 mg iodine/mL, 4–5 mL/s) ● Delayed scan after 3–5 minutes increases sensitivity where the early phase is negative ● *Caution:* Oral contrast administration is contraindicated ● Detection threshold for bleeding is about 0.5–1 mL/min.

Fig. 5.20 a, b Acute lower gastrointestinal bleeding. CTA showing contrast extravasation (arrow) from a diverticulum (arrowhead) in the cecum (**a**). Coronal MIP identifies the ileocolic artery (arrow) as the arterial feeder (**b**).

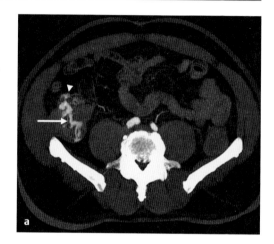

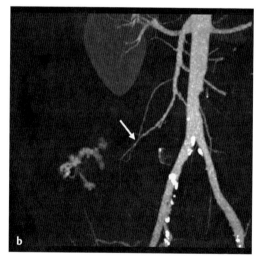

▶ **DSA findings**

Directly visualizes bleeding and the arterial branch supplying it ● Occasionally can indirectly demonstrate the source of intermittent bleeding by visualizing abnormal vessels (tumors, inflammation) or a prematurely filling vein (angiodysplasia) ● Technique involves long image series (about 25 seconds) to distinguish contrast extravasation from slow venous washout ● The often limited quality of the subtraction images because of massive meteorism after endoscopy is a problem ● Advantages over CTA include the option of embolization or marking the

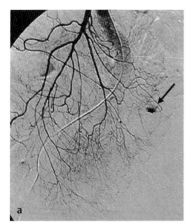

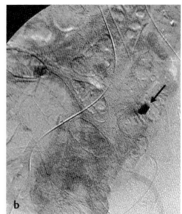

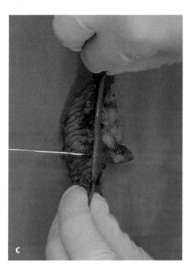

Fig. 5.21 a–c Acute gastrointestinal bleeding. DSA, arterial phase (**a**). Contrast extravasation (arrow) from a branch of an ileal artery in the ileum. The extravasation (arrow) persists after contrast has washed out of the blood vessels (**b**). Surgical specimen (**c**). Source of bleeding is a small bowel diverticulum.

arterial feeder with patent blue or embolization coils for subsequent surgery • Detection threshold for bleeding is about 1 mL/min.

▶ **Nuclear imaging**

Tc sulfur colloid or indium-labeled erythrocytes are the tracers used • The disadvantage is that the poor spatial resolution often does not allow unequivocal identification of the site of bleeding • The advantage is the significantly lower detection threshold for bleeding than CTA and DSA—about 0.1 mL/min • This makes this modality suitable for detecting subacute or chronic bleeding • Not indicated as the initial study in acute bleeding.

Clinical Aspects

▶ **Typical presentation**

Hematemesis (upper gastrointestinal bleeding) • Melena (tarry stool) • Hematochezia (fresh blood in the stool) • Circulatory symptoms due to hypovolemia • Anemia.

▶ **Therapeutic options**

Endoscopic hemostasis • Embolization • Resection of the affected bowel segment.

▶ **Course and prognosis**

Spontaneous cessation of bleeding occurs in 60–80% of cases in lower gastrointestinal bleeding and 80–95% in upper gastrointestinal bleeding • Recurrent bleeding is common • Mortality increases significantly with recurrent bleeding.

▶ **What does the clinician want to know?**

Location of the bleeding • Cause.

Differential Diagnosis

Contrast extravasation mimicked by	– Dense food in the bowel, for example from iron tablets (CT) • Remedied by obtaining an unenhanced scan prior to contrast injection
	– Vessel imaged end on (DSA) • Remedied by using long series until contrast has washed out entirely and oblique projections
	– Hyperemia of a bowel segment, for example, due to inflammation • Remedied by using a lower contrast dose and injection rate
	– Prolonged adrenal parenchymal enhancement due to an anatomic variant with vascular supply from the visceral arteries

Tips and Pitfalls

Delay in ordering diagnostic imaging studies • CT: Use of oral contrast, failure to obtain an unenhanced sequence, no late images • DSA: Contrast dose or injection rate too high in superselective imaging, series too short.

Selected References

Bonacker MJ et al. [The role of angiography in the diagnosis and therapy of gastrointestinal hemorrhage.] Rofo 2003; 175: 524–531 [In German]

Diehl SJ et al. [Negative endoscopy and MSCT findings in patients with acute lower gastrointestinal hemorrhage. Value of (99 m)Tc erythrocyte scintigraphy.] Radiologe 2007; 47: 64–70 [In German]

Ko HS et al. [Localization of bleeding using 4-row detector-CT in patients with clinical signs of acute gastrointestinal hemorrhage.] Rofo 2005; 177: 1649–1654 [In German]

Yoon W et al. Acute massive gastrointestinal bleeding: detection and localization with arterial phase multi-detector row helical CT. Radiology 2006; 239: 160–167

Definition
....

Increase in blood pressure in the portal vein to over 12 mmHg.

▶ **Epidemiology**

Depending on geographic location, causes include chronic viral hepatitis, schistosomiasis, or alcohol misuse.

▶ **Etiology, pathophysiology, pathogenesis**

Types of block and their causes:
- *Prehepatic block:* Splenic or portal vein thrombosis
- *Intrahepatic block:* Schistosomiasis, liver cirrhosis, Wilson disease
- *Posthepatic block:* Occlusion of the hepatic veins (Budd–Chiari syndrome), tumor compression.

Intrahepatic block occurs in 75% of cases ● Most often this is a postsinusoidal block due to liver cirrhosis (alcohol misuse in 50% of cases, viral hepatitis in 40%) ● Increased resistance in the portal venous system leads to development of portocaval collateral circulation ● Esophageal and gastric varices ● Umbilical veins (caput medusae) ● Splenorenal collaterals.

Imaging Signs
....

▶ **Modality of choice**

Color Doppler ultrasound.

▶ **Color Doppler ultrasound findings**

Dilated veins of the portal system ● Retrograde flow in the portal or splenic vein ● Diameter of the splenic vein increases in deep inspiration by less than 30% ● Splenomegaly ● Ascites.

Modality detects possible causes of portal hypertension—signs of cirrhosis ● Budd–Chiari syndrome ● Tumor compression ● Splenic and portal vein thrombosis ● Cavernous transformation.

▶ **Multidetector CT and MRI findings**

Dilated veins of the portal system ● Collateral circulation ● Splenomegaly ● Ascites.

Modality detects possible causes of portal hypertension—signs of cirrhosis ● Budd–Chiari syndrome ● Tumor compression ● Splenic and portal vein thrombosis ● Cavernous transformation.

▶ **DSA**

Now used only for direct portography in a transjugular intrahepatic portosystemic shunt (TIPS) procedure ● Measurement of wedge pressure in a transjugular liver biopsy.

Table 5.2 Normal values for the portal and splenic veins

Vessel	Diameter
Portal vein (fasting)	8–12 mm
Splenic vein	4–6 mm

Fig. 5.22 a, b Direct portography (**a**) prior to implantation of TIPS. Large-caliber splenic vein with filling of fundus varices. Findings after implantation of the TIPS (**b**) and embolization of the varices.

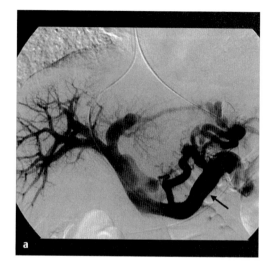

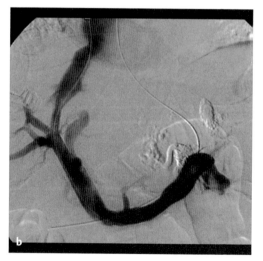

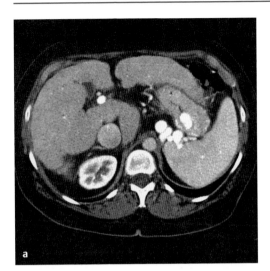

Fig. 5.23 a, b Multidetector CT, portal venous phase. Liver cirrhosis and portal hypertension with fundus varices (**a**), ascites (**b**), and severe esophageal varices.

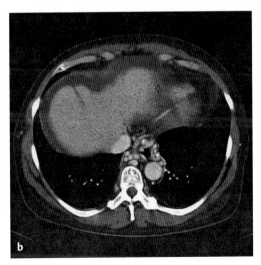

Clinical Aspects

▶ **Typical presentation**
Ascites • Splenomegaly • Coagulation disorder • Caput medusae • Acute gastrointestinal bleeding (esophageal and gastric varices) • Liver failure.

▶ **Therapeutic options**
Treatment of the underlying disorder • Medical, endoscopic, interventional (TIPS), or surgical control of variceal bleeding.

▶ **Course and prognosis**
This depends on the underlying disorder and liver insufficiency according to the CTP (Child–Turcotte–Pugh) or MELD (model for end-stage liver disease) scores • Often chronically progressive.

▶ **What does the clinician want to know?**
Causes of portal hypertension • Vascular topography.

Differential Diagnosis

Congestive heart failure	– Vena cava and hepatic veins are dilated in addition to the portal vein
	– Hepatomegaly
	– Ascites

Selected References

Brancatelli G et al. Cirrhosis: CT and MR imaging evaluation. Eur J Radiol 2007; 61: 57–69

Kurz AK, Blum HE. [Duplexsonography of the liver: state-of-the-art and perspectives.] Dtsch Med Wochenschr 2006; 131: 1035–1039 [In German]

Pieters PC et al. Evaluation of the portal venous system: complementary roles of invasive and noninvasive imaging strategies. RadioGraphics 1997; 17: 879–895

Definition

▶ **Epidemiology**
Found in 0.05–0.5% of autopsies • 1–15% of patients with liver cirrhosis develop portal vein thrombosis • Occurrence correlates with the stage of the disease according to the CTP (Child–Turcotte–Pugh) classification.

▶ **Etiology, pathophysiology, pathogenesis**
Slowed blood flow or stasis in the portal venous system • Hypercoagulability • Thrombus formation in the portal vein can propagate into the intrahepatic branches and/or mesenteric veins • Liver cirrhosis • Myeloproliferative syndrome • Deficiency of plasma factors inhibiting coagulation • Intraabdominal infection (umbilical vein infection in newborns) • Pancreatitis • Pancreatic carcinoma • Hepatocellular carcinoma • Paraneoplastic syndrome • Trauma • Abdominal surgery.
Cavernous transformation often occurs over a period of weeks to months, with formation of threadlike collaterals in the porta hepatis and shrinkage of the occluded portal vein.

Imaging Signs

▶ **Modality of choice**
CT, MRI, and color Doppler ultrasound where acoustic conditions are favorable.

▶ **Color Doppler ultrasound findings**
Acute thrombi on B-mode ultrasound appear hypoechoic and are therefore difficult to detect • Chronic thrombi (several weeks old) are usually hyperechoic • Color images show a flow defect in the portal vein • The resistance index in the hepatic artery is reduced • Portosystemic collaterals • There may be retrograde flow in the intrahepatic branches of the portal vein, portions of the splenic vein, and superior mesenteric vein • Splenomegaly • Ascites • Signs of liver cirrhosis may be present.

▶ **CT and MRI findings**
Filling defect in the portal vein • Portosystemic collaterals • Splenomegaly • Ascites • Signs of liver cirrhosis may be present.

Clinical Aspects

▶ **Typical presentation**
Highly variable picture • Often asymptomatic • Most common clinical manifestations include bleeding from esophageal varices • Nausea, vomiting • Pain in the right upper abdomen • Transient ascites • Hypersplenism • Thromboses beginning in the mesenteric veins often lead to venous mesenteric infarction.

▶ **Therapeutic options**
Anticoagulation • TIPS and local thrombolysis or mechanical recanalization may be indicated • Management of complications such as bleeding from esophageal varices.

Fig. 5.24 a–c   Portal vein thrombosis. CT after contrast administration. Acute thrombus in the portal vein (**a**; arrow) extending into the superior mesenteric vein (**b**; forked arrow). Liver cirrhosis, splenomegaly, ascites, esophageal varices (**c**).

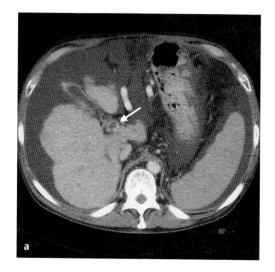

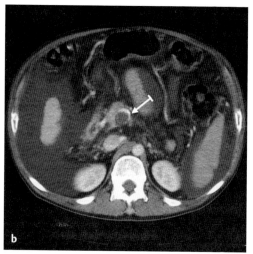

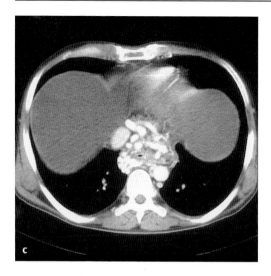

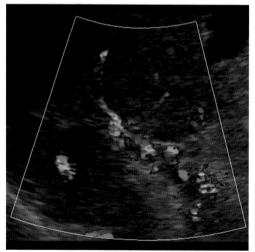

Fig. 5.25 Color Doppler ultrasound. Cavernous transformation in chronic disease.

► **Course and prognosis**

Spontaneous remission from autolysis is rare ● Remission may occur under anticoagulant therapy ● Persistent thrombosis causes chronic portal hypertension and exacerbates an existing condition ● 10-year survival rate is 38–60% in adults ● Cause of death is usually the underlying disorder ● Prognosis is more favorable in children.

► **What does the clinician want to know?**

Extent of the thrombosis ● Cause ● Signs of portal hypertension.

Differential Diagnosis

Tumor thrombus in hepatocellular carcinoma	– Contrast enhancement in the tumor thrombus – Demonstrated hepatocellular carcinoma
Compression or occlusion of the portal vein due to encasement by tumor	– Such as pancreatic or gastric carcinoma

Tips and Pitfalls

Color Doppler ultrasound may fail to detect blood flow in the portal vein due to improper device settings (occurs when pulse repetition frequency is too high).

Selected References

Bayraktar Y, Harmanci O. Etiology and consequences of thrombosis in abdominal vessels. World J Gastroenterol 2006; 12: 1165–1174

Gaitini et al. [Duplex sonography for the diagnosis of portal hypertension.] Rofo 1990; 153: 645–649 [In German]

Hidajat N et al. Portal vein thrombosis: etiology, diagnostic strategy, therapy and management. Vasa 2005; 34: 81–92

Wang JT et al. Portal vein thrombosis. Hepatobiliary Pancreat Dis Int 2005; 4: 515–518

Definition

▶ **Epidemiology**
Rare disorder without a peak age of occurrence ● Females are affected more often than males ● 6% of patients with myeloproliferative syndrome are found at autopsy to have Budd–Chiari syndrome.

▶ **Etiology, pathophysiology, pathogenesis**
Obstruction of the venous outflow tract of the liver at the level of the peripheral or central hepatic veins, inferior vena cava, and/or right atrium ● Venous stasis in the liver ● Swelling of the liver ● Centrilobular parenchymal necrosis ● Portal hypertension ● Regeneration nodules develop later ● The caudate lobe is usually not affected and therefore exhibits compensatory hypertrophy ● Simultaneous portal vein thrombosis is present in 20% of all cases ● Most common cause is myeloproliferative syndrome ● Membranous "web" in the inferior vena cava ● Oral contraceptives ● Pregnancy ● Deficiency of plasma factors inhibiting coagulation ● Paroxysmal nocturnal hemoglobinuria ● Behçet disease ● Compression or occlusion due to tumor (hepatocellular carcinoma, renal cell carcinoma).

Imaging Signs

▶ **Modality of choice**
CT ● Color Doppler ultrasound.

▶ **Ultrasound, color Doppler ultrasound findings**
Hepatic veins are narrowed or not identifiable ● Weakened or absent hepatopetal flow signal ● No venous contrast filling ● Reduced or retrograde flow in the portal vein ● Intrahepatic collaterals in chronic disease ● Hepatomegaly ● Enlargement of the caudate lobe and dilation of its veins to 3 mm and more ● Ascites and splenomegaly are sequelae of portal hypertension.

▶ **CT findings**
No contrast filling of hepatic veins ● Veins may not be identifiable due to parenchymal swelling ● Contrast filling of the inferior vena cava may also fail to occur ● Inhomogeneous, predominantly central, and reduced overall enhancement in the hepatic parenchyma ● Hypertrophy of the caudate lobe with possible obstruction of the inferior vena cava ● Intrahepatic collaterals and hypervascularized regeneration nodules are found in chronic disease ● Signs of portal hypertension.

▶ **MRI findings**
T2-weighted sequences show an inhomogeneous increase in signal intensity in the peripheral portions of the liver ● Otherwise findings are identical to CT.

▶ **Venography findings**
Occlusion or subtotal thrombosis of the hepatic veins and occasionally the inferior vena cava as well ● Fine network of small intrahepatic collaterals ("spider web" pattern) ● Hepatic veins may exhibit stenosis near their junctions or a web may partially occlude the inferior vena cava ● Enlargement of the caudate lobe may cause compression of the inferior vena cava.

Fig. 5.26 a–c Budd–Chiari syndrome. CT, portal venous phase. Thrombosis of all major hepatic veins (arrowheads) and the inferior vena cava (arrow). Inhomogeneously reduced enhancement in the liver, hypertrophy of the caudate lobe (asterisk), and ascites. Anterior displacement of the inferior vena cava due to massive swelling of the liver.

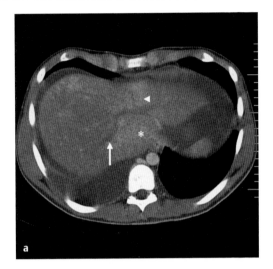

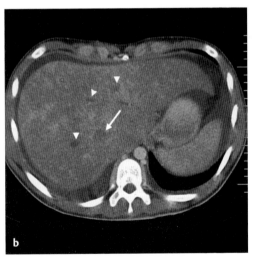

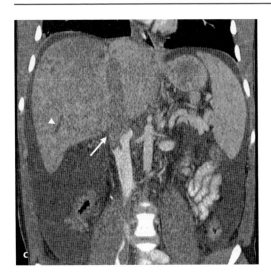

Clinical Aspects

▶ **Typical presentation**
  Upper abdominal pain ● Hepatomegaly ● Ascites ● Jaundice ● Fulminant forms
  lead to acute liver failure ● Initially asymptomatic insidious forms lead to slow
  development of portal hypertension and liver cirrhosis.

▶ **Therapeutic options**
  Anticoagulation ● Severe cases require percutaneous transluminal angioplasty
  of the hepatic veins and/or inferior vena cava, combined with transjugular intrahepatic portosystemic shunt ● Transplantation is indicated in liver failure.

▶ **Course and prognosis**
  Left untreated, the disorder leads to liver cirrhosis and chronic portal hyperten-
  sion ● Fulminant course with acute liver failure can occur within a few hours ●
  Prognosis is good after successful therapy.

▶ **What does the clinician want to know?**
  Extent of the thrombosis ● Involvement of the inferior vena cava ● Condition of
  the hepatic parenchyma (contrast enhancement) ● Signs of portal hypertension.

Differential Diagnosis

Hepatic venous occlusive disease (sinusoidal obstruction syndrome)	– Vascular occlusion at the level of the sinusoids, central veins, and hepatic venules – The large hepatic veins visualized on imaging studies remain patent – Usually occurs about three weeks after bone marrow transplantation
Right heart failure	– Hepatic congestion with dilated hepatic veins and delayed contrast enhancement

Tips and Pitfalls

Color Doppler ultrasound may fail to detect blood flow in the hepatic veins and inferior vena cava where these vessels lie too far distal (especially in ascites) or due to improper device settings (occurs where pulse repetition frequency is too high) ● Where CT portal venous phase sequences are obtained too early, the lack of venous filling can mimic hepatic vein thrombosis (especially in heart failure).

Selected References

Bayraktar Y, Harmanci O. Etiology and consequences of thrombosis in abdominal vessels. World J Gastroenterol 2006; 12: 1165–1174

Brancatelli G et al. Budd–Chiari syndrome: spectrum of imaging findings. AJR Am J Roentgenol 2007; 188: 168–176

Erden A. Budd–Chiari syndrome: a review of imaging findings. Eur J Radiol 2007; 61: 44–56

Menon KV et al. The Budd–Chiari syndrome. N Engl J Med 2004; 350: 578–585

Garcia–Pagán JC et al. TIPS for Budd–Chiari syndrome: long-term results and prognostics factors in 124 patients. Gastroenterology 2008; 135: 808–815

Definition

▶ **Epidemiology**
Much less common than deep venous thrombosis in the lower extremity (ratio of 1–2 : 100).
▶ **Etiology, pathophysiology, pathogenesis**
Ascending venous thrombosis in the pelvis and lower extremity ● Mass or inflammatory process in the retroperitoneal space ● Coagulation disorders.

Imaging Signs

▶ **Modality of choice**
CT ● MRI.
▶ **Color Doppler ultrasound findings**
Not compressible ● Lumen dilated by hypoechoic thrombotic material ● No flow signal.
▶ **CT and MRI findings**
Filling defect with smooth contour ● Peripheral mural enhancement.
▶ **Cavography findings**
Complete occlusion with collateral circulation or filling defect incompletely blocking blood flow ● Only indicated in interventional therapy.

Clinical Aspects

▶ **Typical presentation**
Bilateral leg swelling ● Prominent veins in the abdominal wall ● Back pain may occur ● Nephrotic syndrome ● Hepatomegaly ● Heart failure ● Symptoms of pulmonary artery embolism.
▶ **Therapeutic options**
Anticoagulation ● Systemic or local lysis ● Thrombectomy ● Stent placement.
▶ **Course and prognosis**
Spontaneous resolution or organization of the thrombus ● Thrombus progression ● Pulmonary embolism is a common complication.
▶ **What does the clinician want to know?**
Extent of the thrombosis ● Anatomic causes of thrombosis ● Pulmonary embolism.

Differential Diagnosis

Tumor thrombus	– Tumor infiltration into the inferior vena cava (in renal cell carcinoma, hepatocellular carcinoma, adrenal cortical carcinoma) or primary intraluminal tumor (leiomyosarcoma).
	– Central contrast enhancement

Fig. 5.27 a, b Acute thrombosis of the inferior vena cava. CT after contrast administration. Coronal reformation along the inferior vena cava (**a**) and axial source image (**b**) through the chest. Smoothly demarcated hypodense thrombus (arrow) in the inferior vena cava (**a**) extending continuously all the way into the right ventricle (**b**). Other findings include a thrombus along the wall of the right atrium (forked arrow).

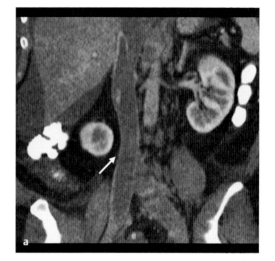

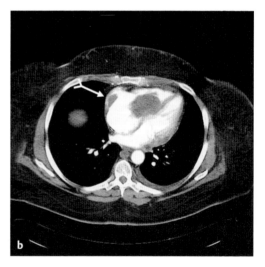

Tips and Pitfalls

Flow phenomena in the inferior vena cava can be misinterpreted as thrombosis.

Selected References

Lin J et al. Vena cava 3D contrast-enhanced MR venography: a pictorial review. Cardiovasc Intervent Radiol 2005; 28: 795–805

Zhang L et al. Spectrum of the inferior vena cava: MDCT findings. Abdom Imaging 2007; 32: 495–503

Definition

▶ **Epidemiology**
Atherosclerosis of the renal arteries is the cause of hypertension in about 5% of all cases ● This is the third most common cause of kidney failure after diabetes mellitus and hypertension ● *Prevalence:* 15% of stroke patients (autopsy finding); 25% of patients undergoing coronary angiography; 30% of all dialysis patients over 60 years; over 30% of patients with hypertension poorly controlled by medication; 50% of patients undergoing DSA for peripheral arterial occlusive disease ● Probability of occurrence correlates with the severity of peripheral arterial occlusive disease ● Atherosclerotic stenosis of the renal arteries often occurs as ostial stenosis. *Fibromuscular dysplasia:* Incidence in hypertensive adolescents is 70% ● Ratio of females to males is 4 : 1 ● Occurs bilaterally in 60% of cases.

▶ **Etiology, pathophysiology, pathogenesis**
– *Below age 40:* Fibromuscular dysplasia ● Atherosclerosis ● Vasculitis.
– *Over age 40:* Atherosclerosis (70%) ● Fibromuscular dysplasia ● Compression ● Aneurysms ● Tumor compression.
Above 70% narrowing of the lumen, an increase in renin and angiotensin II occurs with hypertension ● In chronic disease, volume overload occurs due to hyperaldosteronism.

Imaging Signs

▶ **Modality of choice**
Color Doppler ultrasound ● MRA ● CTA ● DSA.

▶ **General findings**
Size difference between the kidneys (> 1.5 cm in 60% of patients with unilateral stenosis) ● Narrowing of the lumen of renal arteries compared with the segments proximal and distal to the lesion ● Poststenotic dilation is a sign of high-grade stenosis ● Collaterals.

▶ **Color Doppler ultrasound findings**
Flow acceleration in the stenosis ● Poststenotic turbulence ● Color Doppler ultrasound visualizes the origins of renal arteries in only 75% of cases; it is more difficult in the right kidney than in the left ● Accessory renal arteries (present in 30% of cases) render diagnostic studies difficult ● Modality does not allow diagnosis by exclusion ● Resistance index is 1 – (end-diastolic velocity/maximum systolic velocity) ● Revascularization has a poor chance of success where the resistance index is less than 0.8.

▶ **CTA findings**
Arteries are directly visualized after contrast injection ● Rapid data acquisition with the single breath-hold technique ● Pulse-triggered acquisition may be required as renal arteries can exhibit a strong pulse and produce motion artifacts ● Vascular calcification can be readily evaluated ● Higher spatial resolution and fewer flow artifacts than MRA ● Findings are based on the primary images ● Iodinated contrast agent can compromise kidney function in patients with renal insufficiency.

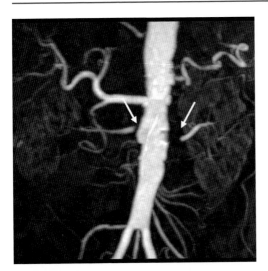

Fig. 6.1 Contrast MRA of renal arterial stenosis as a MIP reconstruction. High-grade ostial stenosis (arrows) of both renal arteries.

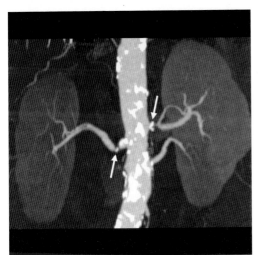

Fig. 6.2 CTA in the MIP reconstruction. High-grade ostial stenosis (arrows) of both renal arteries. Arterial branch supplying the left lower pole is not stenosed. Excellent visualization of ostial calcification compared with MRA.

▶ **MRA findings**

Arteries are directly visualized after contrast injection • Rapid data acquisition with the single breath-hold technique • Pulse-triggered acquisition may be required as renal arteries can exhibit a strong pulse and produce motion artifacts • Vascular calcification is poorly visualized • Stent can produce metal artifacts • Findings are based on the primary images • Phase-contrast and spin-tagging techniques can provide information on function and flow in the renal arteries • Gadolinium contrast agents entail a risk of nephrogenic systemic fibrosis in patients with renal insufficiency.

▶ **DSA**

Minimally invasive • This is indicated where CTA or MRA of sufficient quality is unavailable and where percutaneous treatment is being considered • Used where ultrasound has detected renal arterial stenosis and treatment is indicated.

Table 6.1   Diagnostic criteria—renal arteries

Length of the kidneys	Normal: 11–13 cm
Peak intrastenotic velocity	> 200 cm/s is a sign of stenosis
PSV ratio RA/AA	> 3.5 indicates stenosis of 60–99%

AA = abdominal aorta; PSV = peak systolic velocity; RA = renal artery.

Clinical Aspects

▶ **Typical presentation**

Asymptomatic with up to 70% narrowing of the lumen • Stenosis over 70% causes hypertension • Ischemic nephropathy manifests itself only where parenchymal loss exceeds 50%.

▶ **Therapeutic options**

Treatment of choice is angioplasty with stent • Favorable indications include stenosis over 70% and poorly controlled hypertension, progressive nephropathy (creatinine 150–300 µmol/L), bilateral stenosis over 70%, fibromuscular dysplasia • Surgical procedures are employed increasingly rarely.

▶ **Course and prognosis**

In atherosclerotic stenosis, blood pressure can usually be controlled well with medication • Left untreated, ischemic nephropathy progresses • Occlusion rate of renal arteries at > 60% stenosis is 5% per year • The rule of thumb after treatment with angioplasty and stent is that 25% of patients improve, 50% remain stable, and 25% worsen (hypertension and renal insufficiency).

▶ **What does the clinician want to know?**

Extent of stenosis and occlusion.

Differential Diagnosis

Fibromuscular dysplasia
- Females under 40 years
- Typical "string of pearls" pattern
- Often in the middle third of the renal artery
- Can also involve the carotid arteries, and in the lower extremity most often involves the iliac arteries

Tips and Pitfalls

Insufficient patient preparation (low-residue food, evacuation of intestinal gas, fasting) prior to ultrasound ● Failure to exclude carotid stenosis prior to treatment of renal arterial stenosis ● Treating renal arterial stenosis in the absence of an accepted indication.

Selected References

Garovic VD, Textor SC. Renovascular hypertension and ischemic nephropathy. Circulation 2005; 112: 1362–1374

Leiner T et al. Contemporary imaging techniques for the diagnosis of renal artery stenosis. Eur Radiol 2005; 15: 2219–2229

Riehl J et al. Renovascular hypertension—diagnosis and therapy. Internist (Berl) 2005; 46: 509–519 [In German]

Zeller T. Current state of diagnosis and endovascular treatment of renal artery stenosis. Vasa 2006; 35: 147–155

Definition

▶ **Epidemiology**
Estimated prevalence of symptomatic fibromuscular dysplasia is 0.5% • Prevalence at angiography of live kidney donors is about 5% • Accounts for 70% of cases of hypertension in children and young adults • Females are affected four times more often than males • Renal arteries are affected in 75% of cases; there is bilateral involvement in 35% of these and multifocal involvement in 25% • The internal carotid artery is affected second-most often (25% of cases), usually at the level of vertebrae C1–C2.

▶ **Etiology, pathophysiology, pathogenesis**
Noninflammatory structural segmental changes in the walls of large and medium arteries • Etiology is unknown • Genetic predisposition exists • Estrogen, nicotine, mechanic stresses, and ischemia have been postulated as etiologic factors • Histologic classification is based on the affected layer of the vascular wall, e.g., the intima, media, or adventitia • In 95% of cases, the media is affected and the intima is intact:

– *Medial fibromuscular dysplasia* (75% of cases): Fluctuations in media caliber • Fibrosis and collagen deposition between disrupted smooth muscle cell tissues • This creates a typical "string of beads" pattern where the diameter of the "beading" is larger than the diameter of the artery.

– *Perimedial fibromuscular dysplasia* (15% of cases): Elastic connective tissue between the adventitia and media • This leads to stenosis without dilation ("beads" are smaller than the diameter of the artery • Aneurysm and dissection are frequent complications.

– *Medial hyperplasia* (10% of cases): True smooth muscle cell hyperplasia without fibrosis • Concentric smooth stenosis similar to intimal type.

Imaging Signs

▶ **Modality of choice**
Color Doppler ultrasound • MRA • CTA • DSA.

▶ **General findings**
– *Medial fibromuscular dysplasia:* "String of pearls" pattern of changes in the middle and/or distal third of one or both renal arteries • The caliber of the "string of pearls" is larger than that of the normal renal artery.

– *Perimedial fibromuscular dysplasia:* Smooth tubular stenoses tend to be circumscribed without dilation • The caliber of the "string of pearls" is smaller than the normal renal artery • Narrow stenosing septa can escape detection even on DSA • Dissections in the outer third of the media.

– *Medial hyperplasia:* Focal stenosis in proximal part of the main renal artery.

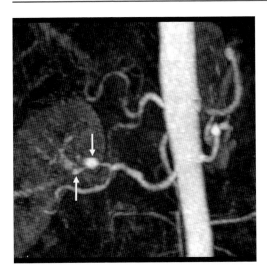

Fig. 6.3 Fibromuscular dysplasia. Contrast MRA (MIP). Fibromuscular dysplasia of the right renal artery. Several intrarenal aneurysms are also present (arrows).

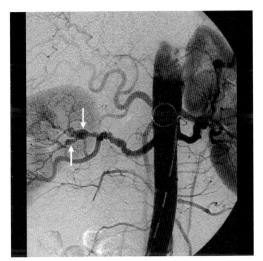

Fig. 6.4 DSA prior to percutaneous transluminal angioplasty in the same patient as in **Fig. 6.3**. Typical picture of medial fibromuscular dysplasia of the right renal artery with a "string of pearls" pattern in which the "pearls" are wider than the normal caliber of the renal artery. As on MRA, other findings include intrarenal aneurysms (arrows).

▶ **Color Doppler ultrasound findings**
Visualizing the middle and distal thirds of the renal arteries is often difficult ● A flank view usually visualizes the artery better than an anterior view ● Flow acceleration in the stenosis ● Poststenotic turbulence ● Modality does not allow diagnosis by exclusion ● The value of the resistance index as an indication of the success of revascularization has not been demonstrated for fibromuscular dysplasia ● Follow-up studies are indicated 6 and 12 months after revascularization to identify any recurrent stenosis.

▶ **CTA findings**
Arteries are directly visualized after contrast injection ● Rapid data acquisition with the single breath-hold technique ● Pulse-triggered acquisition is required as renal arteries can exhibit a strong pulse and produce motion artifacts ● Optimal equipment provides higher spatial resolution and fewer flow artifacts than MRA ● Findings are based on the primary images ● Iodinated contrast agent can compromise kidney function in patients with renal insufficiency.

▶ **MRA findings**
Arteries are directly visualized after contrast injection ● Rapid data acquisition with the single breath-hold technique ● Pulse-triggered acquisition is required as renal arteries can exhibit a strong pulse and produce motion artifacts ● Findings are based on the primary images ● Phase-contrast and spin-tagging techniques can provide information on function and flow in the renal arteries ● Gadolinium contrast agents entail a risk of nephrogenic systemic fibrosis in patients with renal insufficiency.

▶ **DSA**
Highest spatial resolution of all angiographic modalities ● High spatial resolution is important to detect what are often very subtle vascular changes ● Minimally invasive ● Indicated where CTA or MRA of sufficient quality is unavailable and where immediate percutaneous treatment is being considered.

Clinical Aspects

▶ **Typical presentation**
Renal artery involvement leads to sudden onset of hypertension in patients up to age 40 ● Cerebral arteries—stroke ● Abdominal arteries—abdominal pain ● Multiple organ systems may be affected.

▶ **Therapeutic options**
Where there is involvement of the renal arteries, complete recovery can be achieved by revascularization in 50–70% of cases ● Angioplasty is the treatment of choice ● Stent is used only where complications occur ● Surgical procedures are employed increasingly rarely ● Medical therapy is indicated for persistent hypertension after revascularization or chronic hypertension.
  – Revascularization is indicated in hypertensive patients under 50 ● Recurrent hypertension ● Poorly controlled hypertension ● Poor tolerance of antihypertensive medications ● Parenchymal loss due to ischemic nephropathy.

▶ **Course and prognosis**
Worsening of angiographic findings occurs in up to 37% of untreated patients ●
Kidney failure is rare ● Technical rate of success for angioplasty is over 90% ●
80–90% of patients with a history of hypertension of less than 8 years improve,
depending on age ● Rate of minor and major complications is less than 10% ●
Follow-up color Doppler ultrasound is indicated 6 and 12 months after revascularization to identify any recurrent stenosis (7–27% of cases).

▶ **What does the clinician want to know?**
Extent and localization of stenosis.

Differential Diagnosis

Vasculitis	– Proteins in acute disease in 60% of cases
	– Anemia and thrombocytopenia often occur
	– Typical "string of pearls" pattern is rare
	– Often difficult to distinguish from the rare intimal type of fibromuscular dysplasia or from involvement of multiple organs
Atherosclerotic renal arterial stenosis	– Usually close to the ostium without a "string of pearls" pattern
	– Age over 40
	– Males are affected more often than females
	– Typical cardiovascular risk factors
Ehlers–Danlos syndrome type IV	– Often multiple aneurysms
	– Characteristic phenotypic appearance
	– Genetic tests

Tips and Pitfalls

Insufficient patient preparation (low-residue food, evacuation of intestinal gas,
fasting) prior to ultrasound ● Insufficient imaging studies in young hypertensive
patients.

Selected References

Leiner T et al. Contemporary imaging techniques for the diagnosis of renal artery stenosis.
Eur Radiol 2005; 15: 2219–2229

Slovut DP, Olin JW. Fibromuscular dysplasia. N Engl J Med 2004; 350: 1862–1871

Zeller T. Current state of diagnosis and endovascular treatment of renal artery stenosis.
Vasa 2006; 35: 147–155

Kidneys

Definition

▶ **Epidemiology**
Occurs in 15% of patients following placement of a renal arterial stent • Usually occurs within 6 months of intervention.

▶ **Etiology, pathophysiology, pathogenesis**
The acute irritation by percutaneous transluminal angioplasty and chronic irritation by the stent stimulate proliferation of smooth muscle cells (intimal hyperplasia) that can lead to recurrent stenosis.

Imaging Signs

▶ **Modality of choice**
CTA • DSA.

▶ **DSA findings**
Stenosis in the stent.

▶ **CTA findings**
The stent lumen can usually be readily identified with thin-slice multidetector CTA • Intimal hyperplasia appears as a hypodense halo along the stent opposite the hyperdense, contrast-filled lumen • In stents with narrow lumens (< 5 mm) or where the slice thickness is too high (> 1 mm), hardening artifacts can limit visualization of the lumen of the stent.

▶ **MRA findings**
Intimal hyperplasia appears as a hypointense halo along the stent opposite the hyperintense, contrast-filled lumen • Signal loss within the metal stent can simulate recurrent stenosis or make it impossible to visualize that segment of the renal artery.

▶ **Color Doppler ultrasound findings**
– *Renal artery:* Acceleration of maximum systolic velocity in the stent to over 200 cm/s or more than twice the maximum systolic velocity in the aorta • Function of the stent lumen can be compromised.
– *Intrarenal arteries:* Decrease in Pourcelot resistance index to less than 0.5 or a difference between sides of 10% • Pulsus parvus and pulsus tardus with systolic upstroke extended to over 0.07 seconds.

Clinical Aspects

▶ **Typical presentation**
Recurrence of hypertension or worsening of renal functions after an initially successful percutaneous transluminal angioplasty with stent.

▶ **Therapeutic options**
In-stent percutaneous transluminal angioplasty • Procedure may be repeated if in-stent stenosis recurs.

▶ **Course and prognosis**
Left untreated, loss of function in the affected kidney may occur • Repeat percutaneous transluminal angioplasty improves blood pressure and kidney function.

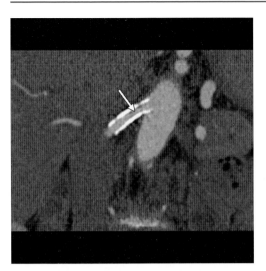

Fig. 6.5 In-stent renal arterial stenosis. CTA. In-stent stenosis (arrow) of the renal artery because of intimal hyperplasia following treatment of an ostial stenosis by PTA with stent.

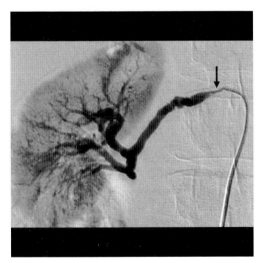

Fig. 6.6 DSA. In-stent stenosis (arrow) in the same patient as in **Fig. 6.5**.

▶ **What does the clinician want to know?**
Existence and degree of any more stenoses ● Kidney size ● Parenchymal loss.

Differential Diagnosis
....

Increase in blood pressure and/or
worsening of renal function due to
other causes

– Contralateral renal arterial stenosis
– Renal parenchymal disease

Tips and Pitfalls
....

Overestimating the stenosis on MRA.

Selected References

Balk E et al. Effectiveness of management strategies for renal artery stenosis: a systematic review. Ann Intern Med 2006; 145: 901–12

Leertouwer TC et al. Stent placement for renal arterial stenosis: where do we stand? A meta-analysis. Radiology 2000; 216: 78–85

Mallouhi A et al. Volume-rendered multidetector CT angiography: noninvasive follow-up of patients treated with renal artery stents. AJR Am J Roentgenol 2003; 180: 233–239

Definition

▶ **Epidemiology**
Most common vascular complication after kidney transplantation ● Incidence is 1–23%.

▶ **Etiology, pathophysiology, pathogenesis**
Stenosis proximal to the anastomosis occurs due to atherosclerosis of the donor or recipient artery ● Stenosis at the anastomosis occurs due to intimal injuries in the renal artery sustained when removing the donor kidney or due to inadequate suture technique ● Stenosis distal to the anastomosis occurs due to torsion, kinking, or compression of the renal artery; improper position of the transplanted kidney; or chronic rejection ● Stenosis over 50% affects hemodynamics.

Imaging Signs

▶ **Modality of choice**
Color Doppler ultrasound.

▶ **Color Doppler ultrasound findings**
Local flow acceleration ● Poststenotic turbulence ● Coarse vibration artifacts ● Waveform is altered with slowed systolic upstroke (pulsus tardus) and reduced amplitude (pulsus parvus) in the segmental arteries.

▶ **MRI findings**
Stenoses can be reliably demonstrated with 3D angiographic techniques (*caution:* Gadolinium contrast agents entail a risk of nephrogenic systemic fibrosis).

▶ **CT**
Iodinated contrast agents have nephrotoxic effects ● Therefore CT is contraindicated in transplant dysfunction.

▶ **DSA**
Definitive modality for demonstrating transplant renal artery stenosis and for initiating treatment.

Clinical Aspects

▶ **Typical presentation**
Signs of primary or secondary transplant dysfunction ● Aggravated or refractory arterial hypertension.

▶ **Therapeutic options**
Percutaneous transluminal angioplasty, with stent where indicated ● Surgery is indicated for arterial kinking, unsuccessful PTA, or inaccessible stenosis.

▶ **Course and prognosis**
Success rate for percutaneous transluminal angioplasty is about 80%.

▶ **What does the clinician want to know?**
Location and severity of the stenosis ● Perfusion of the transplant.

Kidneys

Fig. 6.7 a–d Transplant renal artery stenosis. Color Doppler ultrasound (**a**). Waveform in an interlobar artery showing pulsus parvus and pulsus tardus. The outer contour of the transplant is marked by triangles. Contrast MRA showing distal transplant renal artery stenosis (arrow) (**b**).

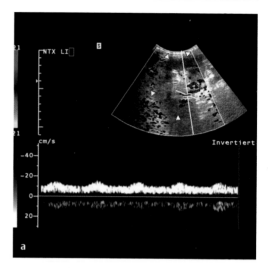

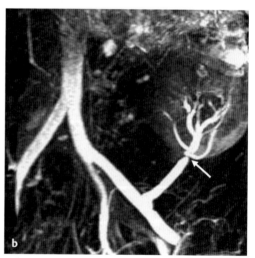

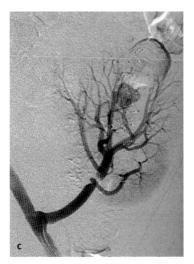
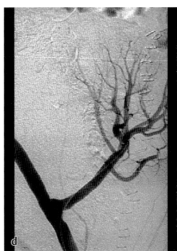

DSA before and after interventional therapy (PTA and stent placement) (**c, d**).

Differential Diagnosis

Transplant renal vein thrombosis	– No flow in the renal vein and parenchyma – Retrograde diastolic flow in the intrarenal branches of the renal artery
Acute tubular necrosis, acute rejection	– Increased resistance index

Tips and Pitfalls

There is invariably a risk of overestimating the severity of the stenosis on MRI.

Selected References

Beecroft JR et al. Transplant renal artery stenosis: outcome after percutaneous intervention. J Vasc Interv Radiol 2004; 15: 1407–1413

Bruno S et al. Transplant renal artery stenosis. J Am Soc Nephrol 2004; 15: 134–141

Patel NH et al. Renal arterial stenosis in renal allografts: Retrospective study of predisposing factors and outcome after percutaneous transluminal angioplasty. Radiology 2001; 219: 663–667

Definition

▶ **Epidemiology**
Rare complication after kidney transplantation • Occurs in less than 5% of cases • Usually occurs in the first week postoperatively.

▶ **Etiology, pathophysiology, pathogenesis**
Hypovolemia • Vein compression due to local fluid accumulation (hematoma, abscess, urinoma, lymphocele) • Stenosis at the anastomosis • Acute rejection.

Imaging Signs

▶ **Modality of choice**
Color Doppler ultrasound.

▶ **Ultrasound findings**
Enlargement of the transplant kidney with loss of corticomedullary differentiation.

▶ **Color Doppler ultrasound findings**
Reduced perfusion of the renal cortex • No flow signal in the renal vein • Retrograde diastolic flow in the intrarenal arteries.

▶ **MRI**
MR venography can be used to confirm the diagnosis.

Clinical Aspects

▶ **Typical presentation**
Painful swelling of the transplant • Diuresis suddenly ceases • Retention values increase.

▶ **Therapeutic options**
Thrombectomy.

▶ **Course and prognosis**
Infarction often occurs with loss of the organ.

▶ **What does the clinician want to know?**
Reasons for the organ dysfunction.

Differential Diagnosis

Transplant renal artery stenosis	– Direct and indirect signs of stenosis such as flow acceleration, turbulence, pulsus tardus, and pulsus parvus.
Acute tubular necrosis, acute rejection	– Increased resistance index

Tips and Pitfalls

The retrograde diastolic flow in the intrarenal arteries is pathognomonic of complete transplant renal vein thrombosis.

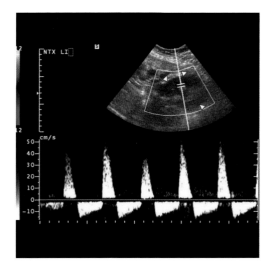

Fig. 6.8 Transplant renal vein thrombosis. Color Doppler ultrasound shows diastolic retrograde flow in a segmental artery, a pathognomonic finding. The margins of the organ are marked by triangles.

Selected References

Akbar SA et al. Complications of renal transplantation. RadioGraphics 2005; 25: 1335–1356

Humar A, Matas AJ. Surgical complications after kidney transplantation. Semin Dial 2005; 18: 505–510

Schenk JP et al. [Radiodiagnosis following kidney transplantation.] Radiologe 1999; 39: 404–414 [In German]

Definition

▶ **Epidemiology**
Occurs in 6–10% of all cases after renal biopsy.

▶ **Etiology, pathophysiology, pathogenesis**
Very rarely occurs spontaneously ● Penetrating injury creates a communicating passage ● Pressure gradient ensures continuous flow ● Often occurs in combination with a false aneurysm.

Imaging Signs

▶ **Modality of choice**
Color Doppler ultrasound.

▶ **Color Doppler ultrasound findings**
The arterial feeder shows slight peripheral resistance and high diastolic flow ● Tissue vibrations and turbulent flow create a characteristic perivascular color mosaic ● This can occasionally be reduced by compression depending on the location ● Occasionally the arteriovenous communication can be directly visualized ● Atypical or arterial spectrum in the vein ● Comparison of flow volumes proximal and distal to the fistula allows quantification (caution: lateral branches may be present).

▶ **CTA and MRA findings**
Premature filling of the renal vein in the arterial phase is often an incidental finding ● Dynamic contrast MRA is indicated where color Doppler ultrasound does not allow a definitive diagnosis ● Very rapid data acquisition is required.

▶ **DSA**
Dynamic examination with visualization of the arterial feeder and draining vein ● Detection rate is improved by using carbon dioxide (for example in transplant kidneys) ● Modality allows immediate therapy (embolization).

Clinical Aspects

▶ **Typical presentation**
Over 80% of cases are asymptomatic ● Symptoms depend on the location and size of the fistula ● High shunt volume can lead to renal insufficiency ● Bleeding ● Hematuria ● Hypertension ● Volume overload leads to heart failure.

▶ **Therapeutic options**
Embolization ● Surgery is rarely indicated.

▶ **Course and prognosis**
Spontaneous occlusion occurs in up to 95% of cases ● Embolization has a high rate of technical success and low rate of complications.

▶ **What does the clinician want to know?**
Location of the fistula ● Shunt volume.

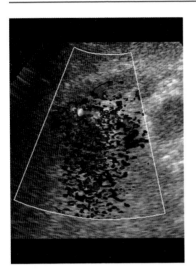

Fig. 6.9 Arteriovenous fistula after renal biopsy. Color Doppler ultrasound of a transplant kidney after biopsy. Arteriovenous fistula with characteristic color mosaic due to tissue vibrations.

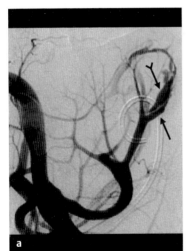

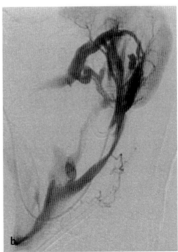

Fig. 6.10 a, b Initial angiogram (**a**) and selective visualization (**b**) of the arteriovenous fistula prior to embolization. Artery (arrow), vein (forked arrow).

Differential Diagnosis

False aneurysm
– Often an associated finding in arteriovenous fistula
– Gray scale image shows an anechoic or hypoechoic area
– Color Doppler ultrasound shows color vortices
– Without a fistula, oscillating flow occurs in the arterial feeder

Tips and Pitfalls

Neglecting to quantify flow volume.

Selected References

Akbar SA et al. Complications of renal transplantation. RadioGraphics 2005: 25: 1335

Begemann PG et al. [Superselective occlusion of renal arteriovenous fistula with detachable spiral.] Rofo 2003; 175: 995–996 [In German]

Davison BD, Polak JF. Arterial injuries: a sonographic approach. Radiol Clin North Am 2004; 42: 383–396

Fischer T et al. [Renal transplant: color duplex ultrasound and contrast-enhanced ultrasound in the evaluation of the early postoperative phase and surgical complications.] Rofo 2006; 178: 1202–1211 [In German]

Definition

▶ **Epidemiology**
Infiltration of the renal vein occurs in 30–50% of cases of renal cell carcinoma •
Infiltration of the infrahepatic inferior vena cava occurs in 5% (UICC stage T3b) •
Infiltration of the intrahepatic inferior vena cava occurs in 4% • Infiltration of the
right atrium occurs in 1% (UICC stage T3c).

▶ **Etiology, pathophysiology, pathogenesis**
Spread of a renal tumor into the renal vein, inferior vena cava, and right atrium •
Spread is usually from a renal cell carcinoma • Occurs significantly less often in
Wilms tumors and urothelial carcinomas • Spread into the inferior vena cava
occurs more often on the right side as the right renal vein is shorter • Histologic
examination usually reveals a mixture of tumor cells and thrombus.

Imaging Signs

▶ **Modality of choice**
MRI • multidetector CT.

▶ **Color Doppler ultrasound findings**
Dilation of the renal vein • Findings include hypoechoic material in a renal vein
or the inferior vena cava • No flow • Low sensitivity for small intrarenal and
infrahepatic tumor thrombi • The primary tumor is usually well demarcated.

▶ **CT findings**
Dilation of the renal vein • Hypodense filling defect in the lumen of the renal vein
or inferior vena cava • Vessels in the tumor thrombus are visualized in the arterial
phase • Infiltration of the inferior vena cava appears as a circumscribed enhancing
area in the vascular wall and surrounding tissue • Images obtained after 3 minutes
usually show good contrast between the inferior vena cava and the thrombus with
minimal flow artifacts • The primary tumor is usually well demarcated • Multidetector CT and MRI are equivalent for measuring the extent of the thrombus.

▶ **MRI findings**
Dilation of the renal vein • Filling defect in the lumen of the renal vein or inferior
vena cava on several levels • Where signal behavior (isointense to hypointense
on noncontrast T1-weighted images, inhomogeneously hyperintense on fat-suppressed T2-weighted images) and contrast enhancement in the thrombus are
comparable with the primary tumor, the lesion is a tumor thrombus • ECG triggering is helpful where the thrombus (which can exhibit a threadlike structure)
extends into the heart • The primary tumor is usually well demarcated.

Clinical Aspects

▶ **Typical presentation**
Involvement of the renal vein is asymptomatic • Spread into the inferior vena
cava occasionally produces signs of venous congestion.

▶ **Therapeutic options**
Resection of the kidney and thrombus.

Fig. 6.11 Tumor infiltration into the renal vein. CT, portal venous phase. Large renal cell carcinoma of the left kidney. Tumor has spread into the left renal vein (arrow) as far as its junction with the inferior vena cava.

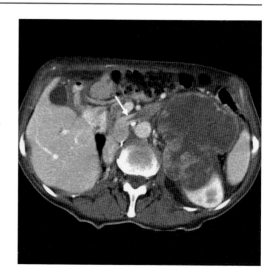

▶ **Course and prognosis**
The extent of the tumor thrombus as a prognostic factor is controversial ● 5-year survival rate is 30–69%.

▶ **What does the clinician want to know?**
The precise location of the cranial end of the tumor thrombus and the condition of the venous wall are factors that influence the surgical procedure.

Differential Diagnosis

Simple thrombus	– Thrombus does not enhance
	– Tumor thrombus is probable where a visible primary tumor is present
Flow artifacts	– Usually caused by slow flow
	– Heterogeneous picture in various phases
	– Images obtained after 3 minutes generally exhibit good contrast

Tips and Pitfalls

Failure to obtain late images to determine the location of the cranial end of the tumor thrombus.

Selected References

Bissada NK et al. Long-term experience with management of renal cell carcinoma involving the inferior vena cava. Urology 2003; 61: 89–92

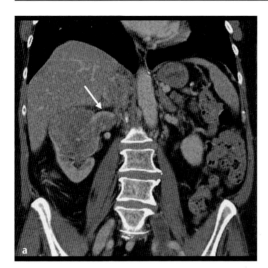

Fig. 6.12 a, b CT, portal venous phase, coronal reconstruction. Large renal cell carcinoma of the right kidney. Tumor has spread into the right renal vein (**a**; arrow) and into the inferior vena cava (**b**; asterisk). The end of the thrombus lies caudal to the junction of the renal vein with the inferior vena cava. Thrombus in the infrarenal inferior vena cava and in the left pelvic vein (**a**).

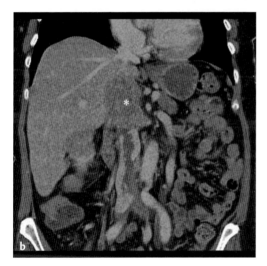

Hallscheidt PJ et al. Preoperative staging of renal cell carcinoma with inferior vena cava thrombus using multidetector CT and MRI: prospective study with histopathological correlation. J Comput Assist Tomogr 2005; 29: 64–68

Kalinka A et al. [Characterization and staging of renal tumors: Significance of MRI diagnostics.] Rofo 2006; 178: 298–305 [In German]

Definition

▶ **Epidemiology**
Cerebral, peripheral, and cardiac vascular disorders are the most common disorders in industrialized countries, accounting for over 50% of all disease • Incidence is 500–1100 : 100 000 • In Germany, 2.2% of males and 1.8% of females are affected • Often occurs in association with coronary artery disease (50% of patients) and disorders of cerebral perfusion • 90% of patients with peripheral arterial occlusive disease are smokers.

▶ **Etiology, pathophysiology, pathogenesis**
Atherosclerosis with abnormal changes in the arterial wall characterized by plaque formation, increasing stenosis, and occlusion • Development of collateral circulation • Primary risk factors include smoking, diabetes, disorders of fat metabolism, hypertension, and age.

Imaging Signs

▶ **Modality of choice**
Color Doppler ultrasound • CTA • MRA • DSA.

▶ **General findings**
Narrowing of the arterial lumen • Often occurs at bifurcations • Collaterals are a sign of a chronic process • Poststenotic dilation occurs in high-grade stenosis.

▶ **Color Doppler ultrasound findings**
Dynamic visualization of lumen and vascular wall • Reduced pulsatility • Accelerated blood flow in the stenosis • Poststenotic turbulence and limited spectral window • Ultrasound in the pelvis is often limited by bowel gas and obesity • Visualizing complex vascular courses is difficult and time consuming.

▶ **CTA findings**
Technical requirements include multislice CT • Rapid intravenous contrast injection is required • Visualization of the arteries of the lower leg and foot is not diagnostic in 10–20% of all cases • Vascular calcifications can be readily evaluated • Calcifications interfere with evaluation and image processing, especially in the periphery • MRA is better where severe calcifications are to be expected, as in diabetes • Remove bone for MIP reconstruction • Segments with severe calcifications or stents are best visualized using slices selected according to the course of the vessel.

▶ **MRA findings**
Arteries are directly visualized after contrast injection • Technical requirements include a moving table, special coil, and rapid intravenous contrast injection • Vascular calcifications are poorly visualized • Visualization of the arteries of the lower leg and foot is not diagnostic in 10–20% of all cases • Good-quality MRA may visualize more vessels in the lower leg than DSA • Image postprocessing is largely automated.

▶ **DSA**
Minimally invasive • This is indicated where CTA or MRA of sufficient quality is unavailable and where immediate percutaneous treatment is being considered • Allows selective visualization of the arteries of the lower leg and foot.

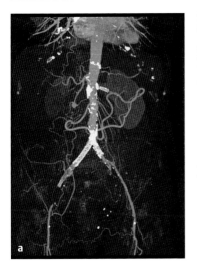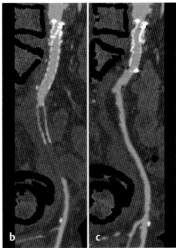

Fig. 7.1 a–c Peripheral arterial occlusive disease. CTA of the distal aorta and pelvic arteries (MIP; **a**). Occlusion of the right external iliac artery (**a**). MPR visualizing the right (**b**) and left (**c**) stent lumen within the vessel.

Table 7.1 Normal arterial values for the lower extremity

Vessel	Diameter
Iliac artery	8–12 mm
Superficial femoral artery	5–9 mm
Popliteal artery	5–8 mm
Arteries of the lower leg	2–5 mm

Clinical Aspects

▶ **Typical presentation**

Intermittent claudication ● Muscle pain with exercise distal to the stenosis ● Pain at rest is usually nocturnal ● Ischemic acral gangrene ● Pelvic type occurs in 35% of all cases ● Femoral type in 50% of all cases ● Peripheral type in 15% of all cases ● Multilevel type in 20% of all cases ● Classifications have been described by Fontaine and Rutherford.

▶ **Therapeutic options**

Eliminate noxious agents ● Reduce risk factors ● Conservative treatment ● Vascular surgery is indicated for intolerable claudication and severe ischemia ● Angioplasty with stent where indicated ● Thromboendartectomy ● Bypass with autologous vein graft or plastic prosthesis.

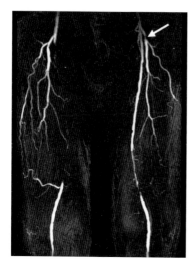

Fig. 7.2 Contrast MRA of the femoral arteries. Well-collateralized occlusion of the right superficial femoral artery and stenoses of the left deep (arrow) and superficial femoral arteries.

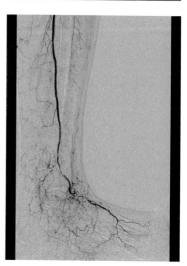

Fig. 7.3 DSA of the arteries of the lower leg and foot. Multiple stenoses of the fibular artery and dorsalis pedis artery, whose branches in the foot also exhibit stenoses and occlusions.

▶ **Course and prognosis**

Patients with untreated peripheral arterial occlusive disease have a life expectancy 10 years shorter than the normal population • 70% of patients die of myocardial infarction.

▶ **What does the clinician want to know?**

Visualization of anatomy prior to revascularization • Inflow • Extent of stenosis and occlusion • Anastomosis sites for bypass surgery • Drainage.

Differential Diagnosis

Monckeberg medial calcific sclerosis	– Structural differences – Calcinosis of the media in muscular arteries – Usually dilating arteriopathy
Embolism, acute vascular occlusion	– Sudden onset of symptoms – Abrupt vascular occlusion, usually at bifurcations – Slight atherosclerotic changes in the vascular wall – No collaterals
Entrapment of the popliteal artery	– Usually active athletes

Fibromuscular dysplasia	– Usually in the renal arteries and carotids – In the lower extremity it most often involves the iliac arteries – Typical "string of pearls" pattern – Remote from bifurcations
Compartment syndrome	– Severe tightening of the musculature in the lower leg increases tissue pressure and reduces microcirculation – Elevating the leg improves symptoms
Venous claudication	– Gradually increasing pain, usually unilateral – Sequela of iliofemoral deep venous thrombosis or edema in the leg – Elevating the leg improves symptoms
Spinal claudication	– Inconstant pain of sudden onset – Difficult to localize, can affect entire leg – Often bilateral, bending forward improves symptoms
Lumbar radiculopathy	– Paresthesias, often in the posterior leg – Occurrence is often posture dependent – Walking and bending forward improve symptoms
Degenerative joint disease	– Joint pain with exercise – No rapid improvement at rest – Pain localized to the leg joints

Tips and Pitfalls

Performing elaborate diagnostic imaging studies without first obtaining a thorough history and clinical findings or where such studies have no impact on treatment •
Insufficient patient preparation prior to imaging studies.

Selected References

Leibecke T et al. [CTA and MRA in peripheral arterial disease—is DSA out?] Radiologe 2006; 46: 941–947

Meru AV et al. Intermittent claudication: an overview. Atherosclerosis 2006; 187: 221–237 [In German]

Meyer BC et al. [16-row multidetector CT angiography of the aortoiliac system and lower extremity arteries: contrast enhancement and image quality using a standarized examination protocol.] Rofo 2005; 177: 1562–1570 [In German]

Norgren L et al. TASC II Working Group. Inter-society consensus for the management of peripheral arterial disease (TASC II). J Vasc Surg 2007; 45(Suppl S): S5–67

Ouwendijk R et al. Imaging peripheral arterial disease: a randomized controlled trial comparing contrast-enhanced MR angiography and multi-detector row CT angiography. Radiology 2005; 236: 1094–1103

Definition

▶ **Epidemiology**
Two-thirds of all peripheral aneurysms occur in the popliteal artery • Males are affected 30 times more often than females • Bilateral aneurysms occur in about 60% of cases • Aneurysms are multilocular in up to 80% of cases • Occurs in association with abdominal aortic aneurysm in up to 40% of cases.

▶ **Etiology, pathophysiology, pathogenesis**
Localized increase in the arterial lumen by more than 50%.
– *True aneurysm:* Involves all three layers of the arterial wall.
– *False aneurysm:* Characterized by turbulent hemorrhage in the arterial wall from an intimal tear (posttraumatic or infectious), covered only by adventitia and connective tissue.
Biomechanical forces • Inflammation with increased formation of reactive oxygen radicals • Matrix enzymes react with metalloproteins, leading to proteolysis in the connective tissue.

Imaging Signs

▶ **Modality of choice**
Ultrasound • Color Doppler ultrasound.

▶ **Ultrasound and color Doppler ultrasound findings**
Circumscribed or elongated hypoechoic area without posterior echo enhancement • Color Doppler ultrasound shows perfused and thrombosed components • Good modality for determining size • Visualization of the outflow tract is limited.

▶ **MRI and CT findings**
Circumscribed or generalized dilation • Perfused and thrombosed components • Suitable for differential diagnosis • CTA and MRA are suitable for visualizing the outflow tract at least in the leg.

▶ **DSA**
Used preoperatively to visualize the outflow tract in the leg and foot • Normal diameter of the popliteal artery is 5–8 mm.

Clinical Aspects

▶ **Typical presentation**
Typically occurs in men over 65 years • Swelling • Pain • Claudication • Thrombosis is associated with peripheral embolisms and blue discoloration in the acral portions of the extremity • Acute ischemia • Patients present with rupture in about 4% of cases.

▶ **Therapeutic options**
Surgery, even in asymptomatic cases • Lesion is neutralized by bypass with a vein graft or plastic prosthesis • Interventional management with stent placement in the popliteal artery is currently used primarily in high-risk patients.

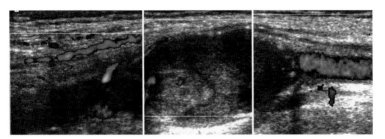

Fig. 7.4 Thrombosed aneurysm with well-collateralized occlusion of the popliteal artery. Color Doppler ultrasound.

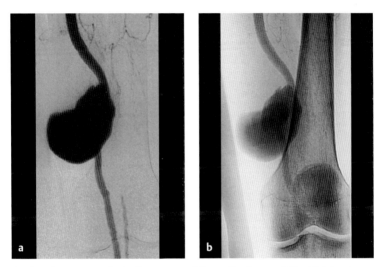

Fig. 7.5 a, b Aneurysm in the P1 segment of the popliteal artery. DSA with (**a**) and without (**b**) subtraction.

▶ **Course and prognosis**
Progressive if left untreated • Amputation rate within 5 years is about 10% • Postoperative 5-year patency rate with venous bypass graft is up to 90% depending on outflow • Two-year patency rate for stent placement is 80%.

▶ **What does the clinician want to know?**
Extent and type of the aneurysm • Evaluation of inflow, the artery involved, and drainage.

Differential Diagnosis

Synovial cyst (Baker cyst)	– Cystic evagination of the joint capsule – Often spontaneously reversible – Patients over 60 years
Cystic degeneration of the adventitia	– Mucoid cysts of the adventitia, occurring in the popliteal artery in 85% of cases – 60% of patients are 40–50 years of age
Entrapment with prestenotic or poststenotic dilation	– Compression syndrome, usually involving the gastrocnemius muscle – Can be provoked by plantar flexion or dorsiflexion – Young men under 30 years
Popliteal vein thrombosis	– Usually identifiable along the course of the vein
Venous aneurysm	– Recurrent pulmonary embolisms in 71% of cases – Four to five times less common than peripheral arterial aneurysm – Usually identifiable along the course of the vein

Tips and Pitfalls

Failure to examine the contralateral side after diagnosis of a popliteal aneurysm • Failing to exclude further aneurysms.

Selected References

Antonello M et al. Open repair versus endovascular treatment for asymptomatic popliteal artery aneurysm: results of a prospective randomized study. J Vasc Surg 2005; 42: 185–193

Rieker O et al. [Popliteal aneurysms: clinical aspects and diagnosis.] Rofo 1995; 120–127 [In German]

Widmer M et al. [Popliteal aneurysms.] Gefäßchirurgie 2006; 11: 299–311 [In German]

Definition

▶ **Epidemiology**
Annual incidence rate is 1 : 7000. ● Peak age is 75–85 years.

▶ **Etiology, pathophysiology, pathogenesis**
Sudden occlusion of an artery by embolism ● Cardiac causes including valvular defects, dysrhythmia, atrial thrombi, cardiac tumors, and endocarditis account for 80% of cases ● 20% are due to extracardiac causes, including thrombosed aneurysm, atheromatous plaques, compression syndrome, and iatrogenic causes ● A rare cause is a venous thrombus via a patent foramen ovale ● Interruption of perfusion leads to organ damage of varying severity depending on collateral supply and ischemia tolerance ● Reduced endogenous intraarterial fibrinolysis leads to local thrombi.

Imaging Signs

▶ **Modality of choice**
Color Doppler ultrasound ● CTA.

▶ **Color Doppler ultrasound findings**
Hypoechoic or hyperechoic vascular lumen ● No arterial flow signal.

▶ **CTA findings**
Complete occlusion of the artery without significant collaterals ● Even in the venous phase there is no filling of supplied organs or only slight filling in incomplete occlusion ● The source of the embolism can often be demonstrated in the same session ● Modality and results are rapidly available.

▶ **DSA findings**
Indicated where color Doppler ultrasound findings are equivocal and CTA of sufficient quality is not or not immediately available ● Abrupt contrast stop ● Absent or minimal collaterals ● Slight atherosclerotic changes in the vascular wall ● Embolism creates a "dome," a rounded contrast filling defect ● Allows immediate therapeutic intervention.

Clinical Aspects

▶ **Typical presentation**
Sudden onset of symptoms ● Complete ischemia is characterized by 6 "Ps": pain, pulselessness, paleness, paresthesia, paralysis, and prostration.

▶ **Therapeutic options**
In complete ischemia, the arterial lumen opens rapidly ● In aortoiliac occlusion, prompt surgical revascularization is indicated as the risk of amputation is high ● In occlusion in the proximal extremities, prompt surgical embolectomy is indicated ● In the thigh or upper arm, treatment also includes local lysis of the lower leg or forearm arteries ● In chronic occlusion and partial ischemia, treatment includes local lysis, percutaneous interventional thrombectomy, and angioplasty after the underlying stenosis has been identified.

Fig. 7.6 Embolic arterial occlusion. Selective DSA of the left arm of an 83-year-old woman. Irregularities in the walls of the subclavian and axillary arteries. Occlusion of the distal axillary artery (arrow). Emboli in the circumflex humeral artery (forked arrow).

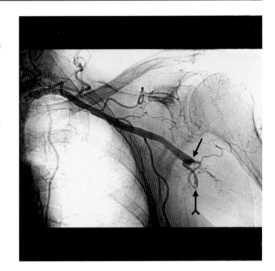

Fig. 7.7 CTA of the left leg. Embolic occlusion of the common femoral artery at the femoral bifurcation. Only poorly developed collaterals are demonstrated.

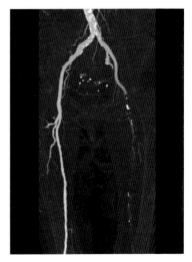

▶ **Course and prognosis**

Owing to the numerous preformed collaterals in the upper extremity, the prognosis for occlusion in this region is better than in the lower extremity ● The chance of saving the limb is 97% within the first 6 hours but then drops greatly ● The 5-year survival rate is 60%, but significantly less with ischemic tissue defects ● Conservative aftercare decisively influences the clinical course.

▶ **What does the clinician want to know?**

Location of the occlusion ● Cause of the occlusion.

Differential Diagnosis

Local thrombosis	– Atherosclerotic changes in the vascular wall and stenosis
	– History of claudication
	– Disorders of hypercoagulability
	– Collaterals, incomplete ischemia
Arterial vasospasms	– Disorders of acral perfusion, usually reversible spontaneously or in a warmer environment
	– Primary Raynaud disease
	– Ergotamine misuse with migraine
Phlegmasia cerulea dolens	– Combination of acute arterial occlusion and venous thrombosis.

Tips and Pitfalls

Delay in obtaining diagnostic studies ● Intramuscular injection is contraindicated because of the risk of fibrinolysis.

Selected References

Alfke H et al. [Radiological diagnosis and treatment of acute limb ischemia.] Chirurg 2003; 74: 1110–1117 [In German]

Definition

Synonym: Pseudoaneurysm.

▶ **Epidemiology**
Occurs in up to 9% of cases after using a transfemoral approach.

▶ **Etiology, pathophysiology, pathogenesis**
Arterial injury occurring in the setting of diagnostic or therapeutic catheterization • Perivascular hematoma communicating with the artery through a pedicle • Particularly prone to occur with insufficient compression after withdrawing the catheter, especially in atherosclerotic vessels • Predilection for the common femoral artery.

Imaging Signs

▶ **Modality of choice**
Color Doppler ultrasound.

▶ **B-mode ultrasound findings**
Hypoechoic mass with systolic pulsation • Thrombotic halo may be present.

▶ **Color Doppler ultrasound findings**
Oscillating systolic and diastolic flow is seen in the communicating pedicle.

Clinical Aspects

▶ **Typical presentation**
Local pain • Pulsatile mass.

▶ **Therapeutic options**
Ultrasound-guided compression or thrombin injection • Surgery is indicated in infection or rapidly increasing size.

▶ **Course and prognosis**
Thrombin injection has a higher rate of success (up to 100%) than compression therapy (60–90%).

▶ **What does the clinician want to know?**
Location • Size • Flow pattern.

Differential Diagnosis

Dissection	– Intimal flap
	– Blood flow in two lumina, usually with different velocities and occasionally in different directions
Arteriovenous fistula	– The high systolic and diastolic flow velocity in the fistula canal causes aliasing
	– Pulsatile arterial flow dynamics with increased flow velocity and turbulence in the draining vein

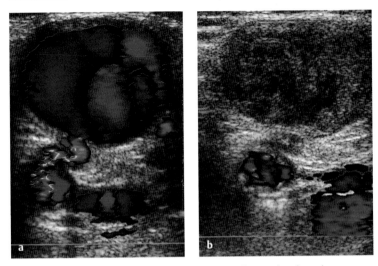

Fig. 7.8 a, b Pseudoaneurysm. Color Doppler ultrasound. Central jet from the common femoral artery (**a**). Completely thrombosed after percutaneous thrombin injection (**b**).

Tips and Pitfalls

Complications of compression therapy include arterial and/or venous thrombosis and rupture in rare cases.

Selected References

Karasch T. [Arteries of the lower extermity.] In: Kubale R, Stiegler H (eds.). Farbkodierte Duplexsonographie. Stuttgart: Thieme; 2002 [In German]

Krueger K et al. Postcatheterization pseudoaneurysm: results of US-guided percutaneous thrombin injection in 240 patients. Radiology 2005; 236: 1104–1110

Stone PA et al. Femoral pseudoaneurysms. Vasc Endovasc Surg 2006; 40: 109–117

Definition

▶ **Epidemiology**
Symptomatic arteriovenous fistulas occur in up to about 3% of cases.
▶ **Etiology, pathophysiology, pathogenesis**
Abnormal communication between an artery and vein secondary to diagnostic
or therapeutic arterial cannulation ● May be direct or indirect (via a false aneu-
rysm) ● Femoral vessels are most often affected.

Imaging Signs

▶ **Modality of choice**
Color Doppler ultrasound.
▶ **Color Doppler ultrasound findings**
High systolic and diastolic flow velocity in the fistula ● Pulsatile, turbulent, arte-
rialized spectrum with high flow velocity in the vein.

Clinical Aspects

▶ **Typical presentation**
Small fistulas are often asymptomatic ● On auscultation, larger fistulas exhibit a
continuous systolic-diastolic machinelike murmur ● A thrill may be also found
on palpation.
▶ **Therapeutic options**
Often no treatment is required ● Ultrasound-guided compression may be indi-
cated ● Hemodynamic complications are treated by ligation.
▶ **Course and prognosis**
Smaller fistulas remain uncomplicated throughout the patient's life or occlude
spontaneously.
▶ **What does the clinician want to know?**
Location ● Course.

Differential Diagnosis

False aneurysm   – Bidirectional flow in the aneurysm neck
                             – No draining vein demonstrated

Tips and Pitfalls

Missing an indirect arteriovenous fistula fed by a false aneurysm.

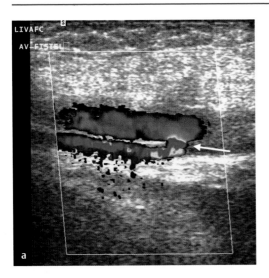

Fig. 7.9 a, b Postinterventional fistula between the superficial femoral artery and vein. Color Doppler ultrasound. Aliasing in the fistula (arrow) is indicative of high flow velocity. Color artifacts in the vicinity of the vein (**a**) due to vibration. The frequency spectrum derived from the superficial femoral vein proximal to the junction of the fistula shows pulsatile and turbulent high-velocity blood flow (**b**).

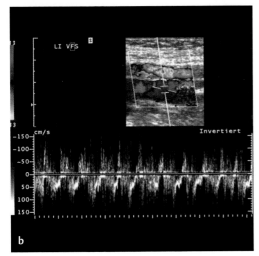

Selected References

Karasch T. [Arteries of the lower extermity.] In: Kubale R, Stiegler H (eds.). Farbkodierte Duplexsonographie. Stuttgart: Thieme; 2002 [In German]

Kent KC et al. A prospective study of the clinical outcome of femoral pseudoaneurysms and arteriovenous fistulas induced by arterial puncture. J Vasc Surg 1993; 17: 125–131

Steinkamp HJ et al. [Catheter-induced femoral artery lesions: Diagnosis with B-mode ultrasound, Doppler ultrasound and color Doppler ultrasound.] Ultraschall Med 1992; 13: 221–227 [In German]

Definition

In Europe, autologous arteriovenous fistula is the method of choice for dialysis access • Usually a side-to-end anastomosis is used • Usually created in the forearm • A PTFE shunt is more commonly used in the USA.

▶ **Epidemiology**

In Germany there are 60 000 dialysis patients • Median age is 70 years • Chronic kidney substitution therapy increases yearly by about 5 % • The patency rate for plastic shunts after 1 year is slightly less than 60% and after 4 years slightly less than 40%; for autologous AV fistulas these rates are 80–90% and 65%, respectively.

▶ **Etiology, pathophysiology, pathogenesis**

Microtrauma and inflammation lead to cell proliferation • Cytokines are expressed by smooth muscle cells, endothelial cells, and macrophages • This process triggers neointimal hyperplasia and thrombosis.

– *Early occlusion of an arteriovenous fistula* (< 3 months): Involves technical problems (kinking, rotation of the vein, shear forces) • Turbulence • Venous branches are preserved • Arterial stenosis • Fibrosis of the vein.

– *Late occlusion* (> 3 months): Involves venous stenosis • In plastic shunts, this often occurs at the venous anastomosis • In autologous shunts, it can occur at various locations:

– Close to the arterial anastomosis due to technical problems or venous atherosclerosis

– At the puncture site due to fibrosis of the venous wall

– Often associated with aneurysms

– At the junction of the vein with the deep venous system or at venous valves due to hemodynamic stresses

– In a central vein due to previous catheterization.

Imaging Signs

▶ **Modality of choice**

Color Doppler ultrasound.

▶ **General findings**

Flow volume in dialysis shunts is 500–1000 mL/min • Imaging studies are recommended at shunt volumes below 500 mL/min or where volume is reduced to less than 20% of the original value • Dialysis problems begin at volumes below 300 mL/min.

Fig. 7.10 Angiography of an autologous arteriovenous fistula with high-grade stenoses (arrows) in the shunt vein. The high resistance leads to retrograde filling of the anastomosis and brachial artery.

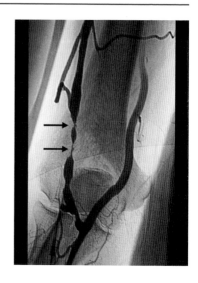

► **Color Doppler ultrasound findings**
 Calculating shunt volume:
 – V [mL/min] = flow velocity [cm/min] × vascular radius^2 [cm] × π
 – Normal monophasic spectrum (continuous blood flow with systolic peaks) • Increased peripheral resistance (spectrum of an artery of an extremity) in the feeding artery and/or vein is a sign of relevant stenosis • Lumen of the vein is narrowed by hypoechoic material along the wall • Findings in an older autologous shunt include relative stenosis with accelerated flow at the anastomosis • Poststenotic turbulence due to dilation of the artery and vein are not relevant per se • Stenosis is quantified primarily by flow volume per unit time • Aneurysms in the shunt are well visualized • Central veins are visualized only to a limited extent.

► **Multidetector CT and MRI**
 Usually not required for evaluating the arteriovenous fistula • Well suited for evaluating central venous stenosis.

► **DSA findings**
 Can be performed quickly and easily via the dialysis access port after dialysis • Retrograde visualization of the artery involves suprasystolic proximal stasis • Visualization via arterial access is an alternative • Well suited for evaluating central drainage • Allows immediate intervention.

Clinical Aspects

▶ **Typical presentation**
Continuous hum and flow murmur are reduced ● Strong pulsation indicative of increased resistance.

▶ **Therapeutic options**
Angioplasty is indicated for stenosis over 50% with simultaneously reduced flow volume ● Central stenosis is treated by angioplasty, with a stent where indicated ● Vascular surgery is the treatment of choice for an immature shunt ● For other stenoses, angioplasty and surgery are equivalent treatments.

▶ **Course and prognosis**
The technical success rate of angioplasty in autologous arteriovenous shunts is over 90% ● Primary patency rate is slightly less than 50% ● Assisted 1-year patency rate is slightly less than 80%.

▶ **What does the clinician want to know?**
Measurement of shunt volume ● Position of the stenosis.

Differential Diagnosis

Shunt infection	– More common with plastic shunts
	– Clinical diagnosis: tenderness to palpation and erythema

Tips and Pitfalls

Neglecting to examine the arteries of the arm (often atherosclerosis with peripheral arterial occlusive disease) ● Pulse repetition frequency set too low with a high shunt volume ● Applying insufficient pressure to the transducer head (adapt to filling pressure and vibration).

Selected References

Clevert DA et al. Formen und Komplikationen des Hämodialyseshunts—Stellenwert der Sonographie. Radiologe 2007.

Schaefer PJ et al. [Does interventional therapy prolong the patency of hemodialysis fistulas and grafts?] Rofo 2006; 178: 1121–1127 [In German]

Surlan M, Popovic P. The role of interventional radiology in management of patients with end-stage renal disease. Eur J Radiol 2003; 46: 96–114

Definition

Thrombus in or occlusion of the subclavian and axillary veins.

▶ **Epidemiology**

Far less common than thrombosis in the lower extremity ● High prevalence in dialysis patients ● 20–25% of patients with dialysis shunt dysfunction have central venous stenosis ● Nearly invariably associated with prior subclavian catheterization ● Over 40% of patients with subclavian catheter but only 10% of those with jugular catheter develop central venous stenosis ● About 7% of cases are associated with peripheral access to central veins ● Duration of catheterization and catheter caliber are relevant criteria.

▶ **Etiology, pathophysiology, pathogenesis**

Puncture trauma ● Foreign body in the vein ● Continuous friction from respiratory motion ● High flow with a dialysis shunt ● Microtrauma and inflammation lead to cell proliferation ● Microvascular proliferation ● Cytokines are expressed by smooth muscle cells, endothelial cells, and macrophages ● This process triggers neointimal hyperplasia and thrombosis ● Genetic and acquired thrombophilia is a predisposing factor.

Imaging Signs

▶ **Modality of choice**

Color Doppler ultrasound ● CTA ● MRA ● venography.

▶ **General findings**

Filling defect on the angiogram (thrombus) ● Thrombus organization and spontaneous recanalization ● Stenosis and occlusion, usually with well-developed collaterals and thickening or irregularities of the vascular wall.

▶ **Color Doppler ultrasound findings**

Examination includes comparison with the contralateral side ● On the affected side, the vascular lumen is obliterated during deep inspiration and atrial pulse (be alert to large-caliber collaterals) ● Acute hypoechoic thrombus dilates the vein, occasionally incompletely blocking blood flow ● Stenosis is accompanied by thickening of the vascular wall, turbulence, and collaterals ● Central subclavian and brachiocephalic veins are often not directly visualized.

▶ **CT and MRI findings**

Veins are visualized after injection of contrast into the foot ● Comprehensive visualization of extravascular compression ● MRI demonstrates paravenous edema and contrast enhancement ● Flow artifacts can lead to false-positive findings ● CT entails a risk of contrast-induced nephropathy in patients with impaired renal function ● Gadolinium MRI contrast agents entail a risk of nephrogenic systemic fibrosis in patients with renal insufficiency.

▶ **Venography findings**

Standard according to DOQI guidelines ● Can be performed immediately after dialysis through the same access port ● Requires less contrast agent than CT ● Allows immediate percutaneous therapy.

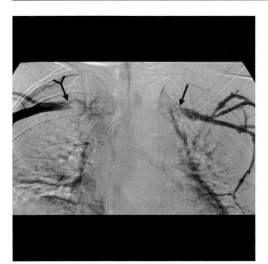

Fig. 7.11 Venography. Central stenosis of the left subclavian vein (here with a pacemaker cable; arrow) and stenosis of the right subclavian vein (transjugular Shaldon catheter; forked arrow).

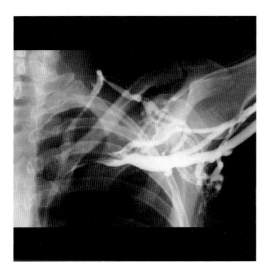

Fig. 7.12 Venography. Central venous catheter and occlusion of the left subclavian vein.

Clinical Aspects

▶ **Typical presentation**

Acute thrombosis creates a sensation of tension and pain • Often asymptomatic due to development of collaterals • Symptoms almost invariably occur after creation of a dialysis shunt • Inadequate dialysis with recirculation • Edema in the arm and chest, collaterals in the chest wall, pleural effusion ● Unilateral brachio-cephalic vein occlusion does not usually lead to superior inflow tract congestion.

▶ **Therapeutic options**

Acute onset is treated by removal of the central catheter, elevation, and anticoagulation ● Pulmonary embolism occurs 10 times less often than in thrombosis of the lower extremity ● Angioplasty is indicated for symptomatic central stenosis ● Stent placement is indicated for elastic stenosis and recurrence within 3 months.

▶ **Course and prognosis**

Technical rate of success for angioplasty is about 90% ● Six-month patency rate is 30–60% ● Reintervention is often required ● After stent placement, stenoses recur later but probably no less often.

▶ **What does the clinician want to know?**

Location and extent of the thrombosis or stenosis ● Cause of any extravascular compression.

Differential Diagnosis

Special type of Paget–von Schrötter syndrome (effort thrombosis)	– Usually active athletes whose sports involve frequent stress position of the arm – Acute swelling, pain, and cyanosis of the arm – Treatment involves fibrinolysis or thrombectomy
Compression of the central veins	– Usually due to lymphadenopathy, mediastinal tumors, or radiation therapy – Usually no thrombosis or changes in the venous wall
Thoracic outlet syndrome	– Compression of the subclavian artery and vein and brachial plexus by a cervical rib, the first rib and clavicle, or a gap in the scalenus posterior muscle (not venous) – Often painful due to irritation of the brachial plexus – Less often involves abnormal arterial changes with ischemia or intermittent swelling of the arm – Provocative tests, with imaging studies where indicated

Tips and Pitfalls

Failure to perform color Doppler ultrasound examination of the contralateral side as well ● Incautious selection of central venous access sites, such as via the subclavian vein.

Selected References

Agarwal AK et al. Central vein stenosis: a nephrologist's perspective. Semin Dial 2007; 20: 53–62

Haage P et al. Nontraumatic vascular emergencies: imaging and intervention in acute venous occlusion. Eur Radiol 2002; 12: 2627–2643

Definition

▶ **Epidemiology**
Annual incidence of venous thromboembolic disease is 100–200 : 100 000 ● Risk of thrombosis increases with age.

▶ **Etiology, pathophysiology, pathogenesis**
- *High risk of thrombosis:* Hip or leg fracture ● Total hip or knee arthroplasty ● General surgery ● Multiple trauma ● Spinal cord injury.
- *Moderate risk of thrombosis:* Knee arthroscopy ● Central venous catheter ● Chemotherapy ● Heart or lung failure ● Hormone replacement therapy ● Malignant tumor ● Oral contraception ● Cerebral insult ● Postpartum phase ● History of thrombosis ● Thrombophilia.
- *Low risk of thrombosis:* Bed rest for up to 3 days ● Immobilization in a sitting position (long car trips or flights) ● Age ● Laparoscopy ● Obesity ● Pregnancy ● Varices.

Imaging Signs

▶ **Modality of choice**
Color Doppler ultrasound.

▶ **Color Doppler ultrasound findings**
Vein is not compressible ● Increase in vascular lumen to more than twice that of the accompanying artery ● Intraluminal structural changes (hypoechoic to hyperechoic) ● No flow signal ● Ectasia of adjacent veins (collateral circulation).

▶ **Phlebography**
Reserved for uncertain cases ● May be indicated preoperatively ● Filling defect caused by the end of the thrombus (contour sign) ● Contrast flows around the thrombus (dome sign) ● Veins show irregular filling or are not visualized ● Collateral veins.

▶ **CT and MRI findings**
Superior to color Doppler ultrasound in the pelvis ● Visualizes abnormal masses immediately adjacent to the vessel ● Simultaneously detects pulmonary artery embolisms (especially CT).

Clinical Aspects

▶ **Typical presentation**
Edema ● Pain ● Sensation of tension ● Cyanosis ● Prominent veins ● Fever ● Malaise ● Tachycardia ● Positive D-dimer test.

▶ **Therapeutic options**
Initial anticoagulation with low-molecular-weight heparin ● Additional measures to eliminate thrombus (lysis, surgery) where indicated ● Secondary prophylaxis with vitamin K antagonist ● Inferior vena cava filter.

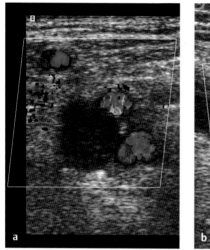
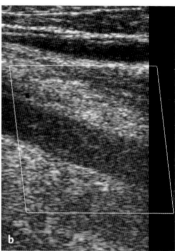

Fig. 7.13 a, b Acute thrombosis of the femoral vein with total occlusion. Transverse (**a**) and longitudinal (**b**) color Doppler images. The image shows a significantly dilated, hypoechoic venous lumen without a Doppler signal.

▶ **Course and prognosis**
Complications: Pulmonary artery embolism • Recurrent thrombosis • Post-thrombotic syndrome.

▶ **What does the clinician want to know?**
Extent of thrombosis • Anatomic causes in applicable cases, such as in pelvic vein thrombosis.

Differential Diagnosis

Hematoma in muscle	– Nonperfused hypoechoic mass in the musculature – Muscle fiber may be interrupted (in a muscle fiber tear)
Baker cyst	– Anechoic to hyperechoic mass in the popliteal fossa depending on the underlying disorder
Arteriovenous fistula	– High-flow fistula (with aliasing) – Pulsatile arterialized Doppler spectrum with high flow velocity in the vein cranial to the junction of the fistula

Tips and Pitfalls

Failure to visualize the distal and proximal margins of the thrombus ● False-positive findings may occur with elevated venous pressure, thoracic respiration, and inadequate compression ● False-negative findings may occur with short thromboses, insufficient overlapping of the examination areas, or massive edema.

Selected References

Ansell JE. Venous thrombosis. In: Creager MA et al. (eds.). Vascular Medicine: A Companion to Braunwald's Heart Disease. Philadelphia: Saunders; 2006

Interdisziplinäre S2-Leitlinie: Venenthrombose und Lungenembolie. Vasa 2005; 34: 5–24

Stiegler H. [Superficial and deep venous systems of the lower extremity.] In: Kubale R, Stiegler H (eds.). Farbkodierte Duplexsonographie. Stuttgart: Thieme; 2002 [In German]

Definition

▶ **Epidemiology**
  Prevalence in the early stage is 35–50%, in the advanced stage is 5–15%, and in
  the stage of chronic venous insufficiency is 3–5% ● Increases significantly with
  age ● Affects 31% of people under 50 years and 70% of people over 50 years ●
  Women are affected three times as often as men ● Other factors include the
  number of births, genetic predisposition, obesity, and occupations that require
  prolonged sitting and standing ● Forms include reticular varices (65%), side
  branch varices (50%), spider veins (38%), and truncal varices (20%); 80% of these
  involve the greater saphenous vein and 20% the lesser saphenous vein.

▶ **Etiology, pathophysiology, pathogenesis**
  – *Primary varicose veins* (70% of cases): Degenerative changes in the walls of su-
    perficial epifascial veins ● Destruction of elastic fibers ● Decrease in muscle
    cells and formation of collagen fibers.
  – *Secondary varices* (30%): Sequela of disease in the deep subfascial veins ● Di-
    lation of the veins ● Loss of valve competence ● This leads to increased pres-
    sure in the veins ● Can spread distally from the junction valves of the greater
    and lesser saphenous veins ● This can later lead to complete varicose veins ●
    The disorder can arise from the perforating veins (incomplete varicose veins).

Imaging Signs

▶ **Modality of choice**
  Color Doppler ultrasound.

▶ **Color Doppler ultrasound findings**
  Modality provides a combination of morphology and flow analysis in the supine,
  standing, and sitting patient ● Visualizes the precise position of the junctions of
  the greater and lesser saphenous veins ● In normal respiratory modulation, flow
  toward the heart is decreased in inspiration and increased in expiration ● Valsalva maneuver shows normal dilation of the veins and cessation of flow, but a
  change in color with reflux ● Visualization of the reflux site and the proximal
  and distal points of insufficiency (classification described by Hach) ● Visualization of tortuous dilated perforating veins with abnormal flow to the epifascial
  veins under compression and decompression ● Modality can exclude deep venous thrombosis in the legs (secondary varicose veins) ● Modality can exclude
  postthrombotic changes in the venous wall.

▶ **MRI and multidetector CT**
  Well suited for visualizing the pelvic veins and inferior vena cava.

▶ **Phlebography**
  Ascending phlebography is inferior to color Doppler ultrasound according to the
  guidelines of the German Society of Vascular Surgery ● It is used preoperatively only where color Doppler ultrasound is unavailable or findings are equivocal ● The
  modality can reliably visualize atypical perforating veins in incomplete varicose
  veins ● Visualizes complex anatomic situations prior to surgery on the lesser saphenous vein and in recurrence after crossectomy ● Allows selective varicography.

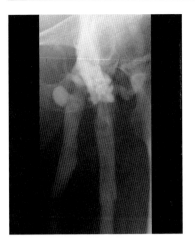

Fig. 7.14 Ascending phlebography. Insufficiency of the greater saphenous vein with retrograde filling during the Valsalva maneuver. Filling of the branches of the venous confluence and a variceal node of the proximal greater saphenous vein.

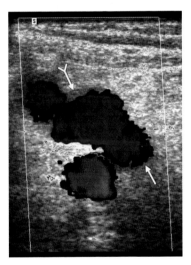

Fig. 7.15 Color Doppler ultrasound in insufficiency of the lesser saphenous vein. Popliteal vein (arrow) and significantly dilated lesser saphenous vein (forked arrow).

Table 7.2 Diameter of veins at the end of inspiration on ultrasound

Vessel	Diameter
Common femoral vein	10.8 ± 1.6 mm
Popliteal vein	9.3 ± 1.8 mm
Proximal greater saphenous vein	4 ± 1 mm
Perforating veins	2–2.3 mm

Clinical Aspects

▶ **Typical presentation**

Symptoms occur in about 50% of patients with varicose veins ● Sensation of tension and weight in the lower legs, especially after long periods of sitting and standing ● Edema in the ankles especially in the evening is an early sign of chronic venous insufficiency.

▶ **Therapeutic options**

Conservative treatment ● Sclerotherapy of superficial varices ● Surgery according to the specific stage of disease ● Endovascular laser or radiofrequency ablation.

▶ **Course and prognosis**

Prognosis for varicose veins is good ● Apart from cosmetic considerations, progression of venous insufficiency with the risk of development of chronic venous insufficiency is a reason for treatment ● Chronic venous insufficiency is progressive ● The goal of treatment is to arrest the progression.

▶ **What does the clinician want to know?**

Type of varices ● Severity ● Involvement of the deep venous system ● Complications of varicose veins.

Differential Diagnosis

Lymph edema	– Normal venous anatomy
Trophic disorders in peripheral arterial occlusive disease	– Claudication with arterial stenoses – Normal venous anatomy
Right heart failure with congestion, impaired drainage in the pelvic veins or inferior vena cava	– Dilated veins – Often continuous flow – Valsalva maneuver does not demonstrate reflux

Tips and Pitfalls

Examining only the junction region in varicose veins (incomplete varicose veins) ● Neglecting to examine deep veins (secondary varicose veins) ● Neglecting to examine arteries (to exclude peripheral arterial occlusive disease in chronic venous insufficiency).

Selected References

Bergan JJ et al. Chronic venous disease. N Engl J Med 2006, 355: 488–498

Creager M et al. Vascular Medicine: A Companion to Braunwald's Heart Disease. Philadelphia: Saunders; 2006

Do DD, Husmann M. [Diagnosis of venous disease.] Herz 2007; 32: 10–17 [In German]

Jünger M, Sipperl K. Erkrankungen der Venen – Diagnostik und Therapieoptionen im Wandel. Akt Dermatol 2004; 30: 407–417

Definition

Synonym: Buerger disease.

▶ **Epidemiology**

Typically affects young smokers ● Males are affected 7.5 times as often as females ● Initial symptoms occur before age 45 ● Common in Asia ● Proportion of all patients with peripheral arterial occlusive disease in western Europe is less than 6%, in India 45–63%.

▶ **Etiology, pathophysiology, pathogenesis**

Non-atherosclerotic segmental inflammatory disorder ● Affects small- and medium-sized arteries and veins in the extremities ● Etiology is unknown ● Inflammatory thrombi occur initially ● Organization of the thrombi occurs later ● Recanalization ● Vascularization of the media ● Perivascular fibrosis ● Segmental involvement ● Usually affects several extremities ● The vascular wall including the elastica interna remains intact ● Acute phase markers are not elevated in contrast to most vasculitides ● Cigarette smoking is essential for the development and progression of the disease.

Imaging Signs

▶ **Modality of choice**

DSA.

▶ **MRA and CTA findings**

Can exclude proximal vascular changes ● Vascular calcifications are atypical ● Can exclude proximal sources of embolism.

▶ **DSA findings**

No pathognomonic findings ● Multiple vascular occlusions with "corkscrew" collaterals ● Distribution: 70% legs, 10% arms, 20% arms and legs ● Usually distal to the brachial and popliteal arteries ● Commonly affects the anterior or posterior tibial artery (40%) and ulnar artery (12%) ● Segmental involvement.

Clinical Aspects

▶ **Typical presentation**

Sensitivity to cold may be an early manifestation ● Erythematous or cyanotic discoloration of the extremities ● Claudication is often misinterpreted as an orthopedic problem ● Superficial thrombophlebitis occurs in 40% of cases ● Late sequelae include ulcers and neuropathy.

▶ **Therapeutic options**

Total abstinence from nicotine ● All other forms of therapy are palliative (foot care, sympathectomy, revascularization with abstinence from nicotine).

▶ **Course and prognosis**

No reduction of life expectancy ● Abstinence from nicotine can prevent amputation in 90% of cases ● Amputation rate in smokers is over 40% ● Number of amputations correlates with social quality of life.

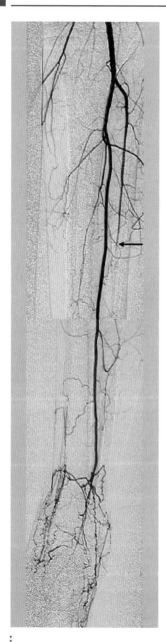

Fig. 7.16 Thromboangiitis obliterans. DSA of the leg. Occlusion of the proximal anterior (arrow) and posterior tibial arteries. Distal findings include multiple tortuous collaterals, which are typical but not pathognomonic.

▶ **What does the clinician want to know?**
Pattern of involvement ● Information for differential diagnosis.

Differential Diagnosis
....

Atherosclerosis	– Typical changes in proximal vessels, calcifications
Autoimmune vasculitis	– Serologic markers
Mixed connective tissue disease	– Serologic markers – Involvement of central vessels
Aneurysm of the popliteal artery, entrapment, and cystic degeneration of the adventitia	– Directly demonstrated on color Doppler ultrasound
Ergotamine, cocaine, cannabis	– History

Tips and Pitfalls
....

Examine all extremities in suspicious cases.

Selected References

Hoeft D et al. Thromboangiitis obliterans: ein Überblick. J Dtsch Dermatol Ges 2004; 2: 827–832

Sasaki S et al. Distribution of arterial involvement in thromboangiitis obliterans (Buerger's disease): results of a study conducted by the Intractable Vasculitis Syndromes Research Group in Japan. Surg Today 2000; 30: 600–605